CURING
PHYSICIAN
MANAGEMENT

CURING

PHYSICIAN

MANAGEMENT

Why Physician

Managers Fail

Alan S. Greenglass, MD

FOREWORD BY

Robert J. Laskowski, MBA, MD

Curing Physician Management
by Alan S. Greenglass, MD

Copyright © 2024 by Alan S. Greenglass

Published by
Winterberry Books
3 Meadows Lane
Greenville, DE 19807

ISBN 13: 979-8-9898930-0-3 (Print)
ISBN 13: 979-8-9898930-1-0 (eBook)

Library of Congress Control Number: 2024901141

Names: Greenglass, Alan S., author. | Laskowski, Robert J., writer of foreword.

Title: Curing physician management : why physician managers fail / Alan S. Greenglass, MD ; foreword by Robert J. Laskowski, MBA, MD.

Description: Greenville, DE : Winterberry Books, [2024] | Includes bibliographical references.

Identifiers: ISBN: 979-8-9898930-0-3 (print) | 979-8-9898930-1-0 (ebook) | LCCN: 2024901141

Subjects: LCSH: Medicine--Practice--Management. | Health services administrators. | Physicians-- Vocational guidance. | Management. | BISAC: MEDICAL / Physicians. | MEDICAL / Education & Training.

Classification: LCC: R728 .G74 2024 | DDC: 610.68--dc23

A special thank you to Dr. Judith Clair, PhD, for permission to use *Why Physician Managers Fail* as part of the title of this book.

Editor: Gail M. Kearns
Copyeditors: Isabella Piestrzynska, Skye Kerr-Levy
Proofreader: Cindy Conger
Book and Cover Design: *the*BookDesigners
Book production coordinated by To Press & Beyond,
www.topressandbeyond.com

Printed in the USA

This book is dedicated to all colleagues, friends,
and patients who taught me not just the importance of
serving others, but how privileged I have been to do so.
Special thanks to MaryAnn Wilson, Robert Laskowski, and
Bob Bycer, each of whom exemplified the values
of helping others to be successful.

And, to my wife and children, who did their best to add joy,
and at times, humility, to my life.

"I think that the whole command and control thing is a relic. It's about engaging people and creating a North Star, a purpose, so that the team is going to give as much as they get. So what's the misconception? The misconception is that you can command and control your way to really creating value in culture. If you want to attract great talent, you've got to create purpose and mission and an opportunity for those people."

—JIM WEBER, *CEO of Brooks Running*

CONTENTS

FOREWORD

You have opened this book and are reading the foreword, but don't stop now because you will definitely benefit from reading this book. The title and subtitle tell you what is coming: all too often, physicians fail at management. This book will help you understand why and also *how* to prevent, fix, or cure what leads to those failures.

Most management books speak to success. The popular management adage "fail often" is used as a mantra of aggressive innovation, rather than a warning about recklessness. "Failure," in current pop management theory, is viewed as a badge of honor—a sign of entrepreneurial spirit. Alan doesn't see it that way.

Management failure is a sign that something is not working; this is hardly a reason to celebrate. No one wants to fail, especially in a medical setting that has important, life-altering implications. Failure can be an opportunity to learn; however, it is often a very unpleasant one with high personal and organizational costs. This book is not a "how to" manual in failure, nor is it an analytic treatise on organization design or leadership. It is far simpler and more useful than that. It is a lesson in humility. Here, Alan relates his experiences and his personal learnings as cautionary examples and the inspiring insight that *humility is a practical management trait*. Being open to being wrong and accepting why is a way to pivot quicker and be right more often.

If you are here, you are interested in management. You may be specifically interested in how physicians manage. But you need not be to benefit from Alan's experience. We physicians often think we are unique, though I will skip over the psychological and sociologic possibilities of why this is so. However, in our self-view of "uniqueness," it turns out we physicians are far from alone. Many, if not all "professionals" (a word that conveys more in terms of ego than it describes an organizational role) believe themselves to be unique. This self-image—whether of lawyers, teachers, scientists, engineers, or sales personnel—creates some specific challenges for anyone tasked with the job of helping them and the organizations to which they belong to succeed. The cliché "herding cats," while apt at times, belies the deeper work of a leader/manager of professionals. Command and control management techniques seldom work with these groups. Respect does. This book abounds in examples of the use of *respect as a management tool.*

One's experiences are generally fun to describe to others, but others' experiences are not necessarily fun to listen to. Personal experience is just that—personal—unless that experience taps into our own. Those who share their management experiences would do well to begin with a disclaimer: "This is my experience. It may help you reflect on and learn from your own." Alan does just that. His experiences and reflections are invitations to the reader to apply the discipline of reflection to their own management experiences. There are many ways to fail as a manager and many ways to succeed. Being self-aware is useful in all approaches. Alan is a great example of a physician leader who has learned and now preaches *the leadership/managerial value of self-awareness*.

Finally, I want you to know this introduction is biased. I have known Alan for over thirty-five years. We worked together for almost twenty of them. I have seen him lead and manage. I have seen him succeed far more often than I have witnessed him fail. Over the years he has taught me much and perhaps has learned a little from me. I know firsthand some of the examples he used in this book. Yet, by reading about them and reflecting on his insights, I learned more about myself. I am confident that all who take the time to reflect on their own work in the way that Alan does in this book will grow as I have.

—Robert J. Laskowski, MD, MBA

Past Chair of the Association of American Medical Colleges Council of Teaching Hospitals and Health Systems; Chair of the Board of Trustees of the University of Vermont Health Network

PREFACE

Is it hard to be a manager, a leader? Probably not in the sense that it is physical or dangerous work. As with many other things we do, at work or at home, leadership and management requires training, practice, focus, and choices. It is often frustrating, tedious, and can feel not worth the time and effort. Often things do not come out right. Sometimes we're not even sure what "right" is.

The intent of sharing my experiences and what I've learned along the way is to help the reader be realistic about what it means to be a health care leader or manager, ideally increasing the likelihood of their personal success, the success of their colleagues, and the well-being of the people in their care.

A number of years ago, a mentor gave me an article by Judith Clair and Morgan McCall published in Physician Executive. "Why Physician Managers Fail" had a lasting and sobering impact on me. I've returned to it often over the years since. When I began to mentor other physicians in management roles, I would share the article. Almost always I got a confused, "Do you think I'm not good enough, that I'm failing?" My answer was "not necessarily," but part of learning, of getting better, is to recognize that we don't know what we don't know.

In this book, I make the argument that medical training and practice often convince clinicians that they know a great deal, and though they may not be infallible, they are at least an authority on many topics. That can lead to blind spots and impediments to learning and improving. I've also shared the article with non-physician colleagues, explaining that I needed them to know the weaknesses inherent in my background so they could better guide and correct me—all good leaders need a team willing to both support and criticize them when needed.

Why did that long-ago mentor give me the article? Probably because I was a prime candidate for failing, which I did a few times, as well as made my fair share of mistakes. I had good medical education, viewed myself as a problem solver, and prided myself as being someone who would use health care to improve the lives of others. I thought management was easy.

This was in the days when it was uncommon for physicians to have advanced degrees in business or public health, before large, professionally managed medical groups were common and before health systems and practices believed in management development. (I was fortunate that my practice believed otherwise). When I was asked about my management style, I answered "to set a good example" and to do what was "intuitive."

Later I realized that warning bells were going off around me. I didn't hear them until I suffered a few setbacks and a bruised ego. But at the time, my bosses and mentor had little choice but to hope for the best. We were a small practice, and there were not many managerial options other than me. Being a good clinician and partner had won me some respect from my colleagues, so I was given my first management role. As you read, you'll appreciate the pitfalls of the selection criteria that got me that job!

This is not a textbook or an annotated research document. *Curing Physician Management* is a practical guide, like a *Physician Management for Dummies* or *The Five-Minute Physician Manager.* It is easy reading and something to return to for everyday practical advice.

This is a book about managing physicians, as well as a book for physicians who manage. Understanding how a physician thinks, how they came to be in their role, will help that physician know her/his strengths and weaknesses, and to correct or compensate for the latter. It will also help leaders and managers better recognize those strengths within the culture of health care so that they can be most supportive and collaborative.

Many of the learnings on the following pages come from other writers and researchers. But the many real-life stories and experiences should have you thinking about how you would handle similar situations—for most of them you won't find the answers in a management journal. Often more can be learned by understanding why an approach has failed than from what has worked by chance. As an acquaintance told me, "Even a blind squirrel can find nuts."

INTRODUCTION
This Book's Approach

This writing is laid out in two parts. The first presents general philosophy and professional styles. What is leadership, and what is it about a physician that might get in the way of being a successful manager and leader? What types of personalities gravitate to health care? How does the training and experience of those people influence how they lead and manage? You'll see each part is broken into chapters, each dealing with a specific principle or, in some cases, a common mistake.

The second part speaks to specific skills. How often have I been told by a colleague that he/she doesn't need to learn management skills? Hopefully, there will be only a few of you who feel that way after you've perused the first part (and you might even find the examples in the chapters on skills in Part II entertaining). For those of you who are ready to refresh your skills, to be reassured of your knowledge and approach, or maybe to learn new skills, we'll talk not only about more mechanical issues, such as meetings and interviews, but also about the fraught nature of critical conversations, change management, and priority setting, among other topics.

A caveat before we begin: No matter how you manage, there will be things that don't work out as planned. There are

No matter how you manage, there will be things that don't work out as planned.

no guarantees. After all, we are dealing with human beings—ourselves and those we manage. Neither we nor our colleagues are perfect, nor perfectly the same, day to day. Ideas that should work with rational people will come to naught if *Star Trek*'s stoic, analytical Mr. Spock did not come to work that day. Or maybe some of the people you work with or manage are more like the volatile Dr. McCoy? You'll have bad days even if you've done everything "right"—just try to remember why you're doing what you do and that, at least in your role as a manager, unlike if you're a caregiver, most days someone is not going to die if you make a mistake.

Throughout the writing, I share stories from my leadership and management career—all true. I've masked identities for the most embarrassing stories, except for my own, to protect the privacy of others. But I have not tried to sugarcoat or excuse how the players, including me, thought and behaved.

PART I

The Big Picture of Management and Leadership
Philosophy, Vision, Mindset, and Heart

"If you don't know where you've come from
you don't know where you're going."
—MAYA ANGELOU

"If you don't know where you are going,
you might wind up someplace else."
—YOGI BERRA

Maya Angelou and Yogi Berra quoted in a book about health care management and leadership? Yes, and the individual quotes seem to be pointing to one greater thought.

We often take note of what qualities have led someone to success in their personal and professional lives. Not as often do we consider how learnings and experiences, sometimes the very same ones, may have contributed to lack of success, to failures. Similarly, many people will not give much thought to what they want to do, what they want to become, who they want to be, and how they plan to get there. In Part I we'll talk about how a person might get to health care management and what helps, and hinders, their success.

ONE

Management, Leadership, and Supervision—*What's in a Name?*

Are "management" and "leadership" just different terms for the same thing? Well, sometimes, and sometimes not. To me, one is often nested within the other. Each function contains elements of the others, and as someone progresses along the continuum (as individuals often do) from supervisor to manager to leader, new tasks and dynamics are added, while others fall away or are delegated.

The legendary basketball player and United States Senator Bill Bradley wrote in his book, *Values of the Game*,[1] that "leadership means getting people to think, believe, see, and do what they might not have without you." He further refers to the even more legendary basketball coach Phil Jackson, saying that to Phil, "The key leadership function for a coach in the pros is getting the players to commit to something bigger than themselves." On the other hand, Casey Stengel,[2] the iconic Hall of Fame manager of the New York Yankees, is said to have had this mantra: "Finding good players is easy. Getting them to play as a team is another story. The key to being a good manager is keeping the people who hate me away from those who are still undecided."

Although we shouldn't idolize sports figures by thinking them experts in all matters (you could say the same about physicians), I think these thoughts capture a lot of how leadership is put into play on a daily basis. Putting aside Casey Stengel's tongue-in-cheek thoughts, a would-be leader could do worse than adopt these and other commonly stated definitions.

But to be more succinct and more memorable—as discussed by Carl Larson and Frank LaFasto in their book *TeamWork*[3]—to me, a leader is *someone who helps others be successful.* As the Talmud says, "Everything else is commentary." All that other stuff—visioning, coaching, example-setting, decision-making, communication, strategizing—are the skills that help the leader to help others be successful.

Then what about management versus supervision? For our definition, let's say that ideally, managers are those people who implement the strategies, plans, and visions of leadership. Managers bring feedback on how things really work back to, and thus influence, leaders and their decisions. Managers will determine the rules and relationships, the policies and procedures, the systems, the short-term and mid-range goals that comprise the road map for the vision and the long-term goals of the group, team, and organization.

The supervisor makes sure the rules are followed and is the one closest to the staff and the customers. Importantly, she/he should be part of the leadership-management team—if supervisors don't understand what leadership is trying to achieve, they can't interpret that for the staff, they can't effectively implement, and they can't recommend fixes. By seeing how rules and policies actually work for the staff and the customers (e.g., patients or other work units), supervisors provide the feedback loop that allows for real-time adjustments or wholesale changes in direction.

Can the same person be the leader, manager, and supervisor? Yes, especially in small or young organizations that don't need or can't afford layers of management. In addition, it is often good for the leader to have learned the organization—or to have developed his/her skills—by having passed through staff, supervisory, and management roles.

There is also something to be said for those who direct the organization to have experienced it as a customer. We've heard about secret shopper programs, and they may be fine as an ongoing tool, but I'm thinking of something else: I've heard many physicians say they became better at their job after they or a family member had to navigate

Managers will determine the rules and relationships, the policies and procedures, the systems, the short-term and mid-range goals that comprise the road map for the vision and the long-term goals of the group, team, and organization.

the health care system—when they themselves received care. Such personal experience may lead to empathy for the everyday frustrations people encounter in their lives, or what they may go through to access care in a health care system. Here's an example, which in retrospect may seem humorous.

When my wife and I were having an issue with our infant child who was unable to sleep without coming into our bed, we asked our pediatrician for advice. He told us that we should leave her in her crib, and she'd eventually stop crying. He then emphasized we were not failures and this was not easy to do. He and his wife had also recently had a child and he said, "We haven't had sex for months because we can't get our daughter to sleep in her own crib, either." The learning for both us, and for the pediatrician, was it's easier to give advice than actually implement that advice in real life.

I've also found that working as, or with, frontline staff opens up a new window into what we expect from them and how customers experience care. A few years back, there was a new concept in practice management called "open access scheduling." It meant that there would be no, or few, pre-booked appointments in a clinician's schedule. Slots would be filled on the basis of same-day phone calls to the office. Seeing that our frontline staff were struggling with the change in their work routine, I decided to take a few turns answering calls for appointments.

I quickly was humbled by the complexity of the work and by the anxiety and needs of our patients. Moreover, I was often discouraged by the stupiditiy of the rules that management (including me) had created and the lack of initial and ongoing training we had provided for staff. Our idea was that open access would simplify how patients got appointments and how the staff did their work. It was anything but, and we needed to make changes in about every aspect of the plan.

This example doesn't mean a new manager needs to "come up through the ranks," but it does mean there is a need to learn how an organization really works, whether you've worked there for years in another role (e.g., as a practicing clinician) or if you're just starting out.

Having said this, there does come a time for roles to be separated. As the job gets bigger, the leader needs to let others do their work, otherwise she/he risks creating confusion among managers and staff who won't know whom to listen to and will then be unable to make decisions appropriate to their level of responsibility. The detail-oriented, controlling leader will find him or herself mired in work they should have outgrown or delegated. It's one thing to stay aware and alert when it comes to details and frontline issues; it's another to try to manage them. It trivializes the importance and the skill set needed of leadership and management to think it can be done well for long periods of time on a part-time basis.

As a manager comes to share responsibilities with an individual or team, it becomes necessary to have clear understandings of who can do what, who needs to know what, and when they need to know it. One of my management mantras is "no surprises." I'm okay with others handling problems and making decisions, but I want to know what's going on. We'll talk more about how to do that in the chapter on Communicating in Part II.

In many organizations, the leader is the founder of the organization (for example, the senior physician) or is expected to be entrepreneurial, or maybe to publicly represent the organization to the outside world. Jay Walker, the founder of Priceline, is quoted as saying,[4] "Management is the art of accomplishing objectives through others, and that's different from leadership, which is more the art of inspiring others and getting them to want to do things." And, "I've always hired managers to do the job of management, which is no insult at all. It's not beneath me in any way. It's just not my strength. Create things? I'm your guy. Solve unusual problems? Maybe. Dream up whole new ways to approach things? I'm your guy. Manage? Not so much." A good leader will leverage her/his own interests and skills with a team that complements her/him. It may not be, as was in Jay Walker's case, the need to find people who are good at things she/he is not. It might instead be that her/his skillset is better used in other ways.

Aspiring clinician managers and leaders often ask me, "Can I continue to practice medicine?"

One of my management mantras is "no surprises."

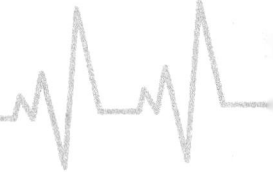

My answer is: "Maybe for now, with well-thought-out support and changes in what you yourself are willing to control. But eventually, maybe not." Why? Because management requires different skills, learning, conversations, and time commitments. If the organization is large enough, and you have progressed up the ladder, both your clinical and management work can suffer. Being able to respond to a management problem in a practice while it's happening is difficult if you're someplace else taking care of a sick patient. Likewise, if you're arguing with your boss for more resources, it's hard to be responding to phone calls about patient emergencies. Being pulled in either direction can not only be stressful but can negatively impact your ability to fulfill both your roles. Even worse, patients may also suffer from your limited availability and attention, especially if they are relying solely upon you and not on a well-functioning clinical team.

A strong team structure can keep you going for some time. The value of knowing (and your patients knowing) that your partners and staff will care for your patients well and will keep you involved and informed when appropriate cannot be overstated. There was a time when I returned from a management trip to learn that one of my patients had been hospitalized and died. I didn't think I could have made a difference in her outcome, but I sure would have liked to have been there to support the family. That episode helped me know it was time for me to stop being a primary care clinician. I knew I shouldn't be practicing even urgent care when I spent more time reading management journals than staying up to date on medical literature and advances.

Having said this, my view is that the ideal for a physician manager would be to keep the opportunity to teach or mentor in clinical situations. That way you can maintain credibility with other clinicians (not be viewed as a "suit") and also maintain the knowledge of how health care is changing, what challenges your staff are facing, and what your practice looks like to your patients. And you can maintain that excitement, curiosity, and caring that was likely a big part of what first attracted you to health care.

MANAGEMENT, LEADERSHIP, AND SUPERVISION TAKEAWAYS

- Leadership and management are not the same but often overlap. There is some difference in the skills needed for the roles.

- Can physician managers continue to practice medicine? Maybe for now, but ultimately the leader needs to let others do their work so the leader can focus on management.

TWO
More Definitions

Doctors, practitioners, providers, or clinicians? Patients, customers, consumers, or people?

I've been in many meetings during which whatever topic at hand was pushed aside while someone, usually a physician, railed against being called a "provider." Was this really a diversionary tactic meant to distract from the topic? Was it posturing to show everyone else who had the power in the room? Did anyone outside of the room care about what name was used? Whatever the reason, it seems worthwhile to be clear what it means to me and why.

Instead of "provider," I'll instead use "clinician" to refer to the professional who practices in health care. Why not "physician" or "doctor"? Sometimes that is the appropriate name, and then I will use it. But here is something I hope we all can appreciate in 2023—a health care leader or manager will not always be a physician. They could be a nurse, nurse practitioner, midwife, physician's assistant, or even a public health or business professional. If we agree there are personal qualities and learned skills that make for an excellent leader or manager, why can't the person be someone without an MD or DO after their name? The potential value added by a physician to this role is their perspective on the science and caring that goes into the work. A non-physician can bring

If we agree there are personal qualities and learned skills that make for an excellent leader or manager, why can't the person be someone without an MD or DO after their name?

similar scientific knowledge and experiential learning to the role, and a partnership with a respected clinician can help fill in any gaps. And why do we think physicians can only be managed by other physicians (and, at least in the past, often males), unless we are stuck in how leadership and management roles were filled in the past? Two of the best managers of medical practices and of physicians I have known were a gynecologic nurse practitioner and a family medicine physician assistant. They epitomized the concept of helping others to be successful.

Next is the question of what to call the folks who come to our offices, hospitals, and other facilities to be treated. And what about the concept of population health, in which we are responsible for not only those who come to see us, but for a group of people, sometimes ill but often healthy for now, living in the community? For simplicity, I will refer to those receiving care as "patients," to those in the community as "consumers," and to both together as a group as a "population."

MORE DEFINITIONS TAKEAWAYS

- Getting clear on our terms makes communication smoother for all.

- Health care leaders and managers are not always physicians—personal qualities and robust skills make a good leader, not specific letters after their name.

THREE
Why Physician Managers Fail

"Modern American medicine has grown a very big brain without a corresponding increase in the size of its heart."[5]

—BILL MOYERS, *journalist*

GOOD CLINICIANS DON'T NECESSARILY MAKE GOOD MANAGERS

This statement is the impetus for writing this book and needs a good explanation. We must appreciate what it is about those drawn to clinical work and their medical training that might impair their ability to be good managers and leaders.

There is certainly a degree of intelligence and education that allows health care clinicians to pass tests to enter the profession. There is the discipline it takes to focus on career goals that take years to attain. There is the care for others that keeps us able to bear the suffering of others and keeps us focused despite fatigue. There is the analytic and scientific education that allows us to make decisions, often with incomplete data. And there is the confidence necessary to function amidst uncertainty. These are all characteristics that are exemplary.

There are also some counterbalances, some "other side of the coin," which comes along with these valuable attributes.

When taking an honest look at the question of why good clinicians don't necessarily make good managers, you must ask yourself: *Why were you chosen for the management or leadership role?* For many non-clinician managers, in health care and in other fields, the path to management and leadership includes specific training, perhaps a college economics or finance degree, and/or a business, public health, or public administration advanced degree. Advancing on the management ladder involves proving yourself with increasing levels of responsibility, learning, and demonstrating your own strengths, and improving on your weaknesses.

Contrast this with how a clinician is often chosen to be a manager. While more and more people are identifying this role as part of their desired career path, the majority of us come to the role in less direct ways:

Perhaps we were chosen or volunteered with less specific training, with less vetting while we were advancing, and often with less mentorship. Sometimes we were just plucked and placed on the top rung of that management ladder.[6] Perhaps we were chosen because we were good clinicians and earned the respect of our peers. Perhaps we volunteered because we were skeptical of the performance of our predecessor, suspicious of people who were or wanted to be a "boss," and thought we could do better. Perhaps we were asked because no one else would take the job. And most common of all:

we assumed the role without specific management skills (and even were contemptuous of such training), without a full understanding of the organization and job, and without a clear vision of how to succeed.

My own story shows what often goes wrong with this kind of process and results.

I was trained as an internist and joined a small, start-up health maintenance organization (HMO) that was partially funded by the HMO Act of 1972 (encouraged and signed, perhaps surprisingly, by President Richard Nixon). My undergraduate degree was in mechanical engineering, and I had no real-world experience or management training. Yet I believed health care should be accessible and high quality for all and wanted to be a leader in achieving that goal. After about a year in the practice, the chief of my unit left. I suggested I could take over.

Given that no one else was interested, I was put in charge of an adult medicine practice serving ten thousand people. My peers supported me in taking the job because they thought I was a decent person and decent clinician, not because of any evidence that I knew how to manage people, create strategy, understand finances, develop talent, or design systems. When our start-up was taken over (after failing financially) by a larger, national organization, I was given the opportunity to participate in a management development program. When the program's director asked me to describe my management philosophy, I said it was "intuitive." I would use my intelligence (as a physician), my experience (barely three years), my skills (none from formal management training), and my common sense (which my answer demonstrated was limited) to make decisions. Not surprisingly, not long after I was asked to step down from my management role. I was told that my colleagues knew I was "at the front of the bus," but they "didn't think my hands were on the wheel." I was going to all the meetings and understood what was wrong, but I couldn't figure out how to improve the way we provided care. My colleagues were each trying to change things on their own because I had no plan to communicate or implement.

I had failed.

Intellectually I knew this, and, in a way, it was a relief, but emotionally I didn't feel good about not succeeding at something I had wanted to do. Fortunately, I was allowed to continue in the management development program over the next few years. I was also given a role that didn't involve managing people as director of quality assurance for our group (which by then was serving more than twenty-five thousand lives). This allowed me to develop knowledge and skills beyond that of a clinician and to meet and learn from expert physicians from other parts of the national organization. When the physician who took my place as chief failed in his own way, I was asked to step back into the role.

It would be good if mine were an infrequent example. Unfortunately, I've seen it repeated many times, which is why I advocate for an organized and planful way for clinicians to become and function as leaders and managers.

As you read through the rest of this section, you'll appreciate more of why strengths as a clinician don't automatically translate into success as a leader and manager.

> I advocate for an organized and planful way for clinicians to become and function as leaders and managers.

DO YOU HAVE A VISION
AND THE ABILITY TO COMMUNICATE IT?

What do you believe in, and is that why you want to be a leader? Do you believe in health care as a right? Did you come to health care out of intellectual curiosity, scientific exploration, or because you enjoyed the technical aspects of your chosen field? Or were you looking for a good job, prestige, and financial security? Or did you enjoy being with or helping people?

When I was considering going to medical school, I spoke to someone a few years ahead of me in medical training. I told him I liked solving puzzles and understanding how things work. He told me that Arthur Conan Doyle, the creator of Sherlock Holmes, was an eye physician (though said to be unhappy in that profession), and what he brought to medicine was that curiosity of how to solve mysteries by understanding why and how people do things. I was sold!

Clearly the reasons I've just listed are not mutually exclusive; someone can be really interested in the science behind health care, in how the body works, and also be passionate about people and how they can be better cared for. But to the extent that the manager does lean to one or several of these reasons and not to all, or that he/she communicates one or several of these values more strongly than others, will determine his/her compatibility in the work culture. The technocrat, autocrat, or financially motivated manager may need to adapt to be successful in an altruistic, "servant leadership," or community-benefit organization. Likewise, a manager who behaves in a more personal, all-involved style may struggle in a rigid hierarchy that might be found in an acute-care work setting

The vision one has and communicates to others will also influence who may want to partner with the manager and come work with the team. That vision is often a prime reason folks show up to work each day and strive to meet the daily, strategic challenges inherent in health care. Staff want to know why they should work someplace and understand what is consistently valued in their performance. They want their performance to be evaluated on pre-stated, understandable, and measurable criteria that aren't arbitrarily changed. And they want to be proud that their work and that of their organization (the whole and their part) is of value and is valued.

It's one thing to have a vision; it's another to share it and explain it to others. It needs to be directly stated and repeated over and over (some would say "eight times in eight different ways"). It especially needs to be shown by behavior ("walk the walk and talk the talk"). When you fail to meet your own standards, you need to admit it. When a job or challenge will be tough and will take time, you've got to be honest about that.

In essence: have something you believe in—say, health care for all—state that clearly, tie decisions and your words back to that principle, and hold your behavior and that of your team accountable to that principle.

WHAT ARE YOUR PRINCIPLES AND HOW DO YOU APPLY THEM?

Having a vision is the first step; next comes having principles that guide how you treat people and make decisions. This is necessary to making your vision a reality. The principles I use serve as guideposts and as an algorithm for how to think through problems. They follow the work of

Rushworth Kidder in his book *How Good People Make Tough Choices.*[7] Here is what Kidder called the "Ethical Decision-Making Paradigm":

Truth versus Loyalty?

Individual versus Community?

Short-term versus Long-term?

Justice versus Mercy?

I've carried these questions in my wallet on a tattered piece of index card for years, and, when stymied by a difficult decision, will pull it out to help organize my thoughts. Here's an example of when it came in handy: A specialty physician was probably the smartest physician in our group. He was someone who often helped with tough patient care questions. He was always compassionate with patients. But he would sometimes annoy his colleagues with an arrogant attitude. After seeing a patient, this colleague would sometimes say, "I don't know why your primary care clinician sent you to see me. He should have known how to take care of your problem himself." Word of this would come back to the primary care clinician from the patient or a staff member. Despite our specialist being counseled about how he was coming across to his colleagues, he continued to consider their concerns to be their shortcomings, not his. It did become his concern when, at the annual review of all the clinicians, his colleagues voted to dismiss him from the group.

Our group vision was high-quality, cost-effective health care, provided in a highly integrated group practice and patient-centric environment. Here's how I applied the paradigms:

- **Truth versus Loyalty**—He had to hear the truth of his behavior and status. He and I were friends, but I could not just be "loyal" to him and protect him from criticism.

- **Individual versus Community**—He was a great doctor for patients, but he was not fitting into our health care community. We could not consider just his individual needs. The tension here was also between the needs of two communities: the one composed of his patients and the one composed of his colleagues. How should we be weighing one versus the other?

- **Short-term versus Long-term**—In the short term, his colleagues might feel better if he, and his pointed criticisms, were gone. In the long term, we would lose a true expert in his field and someone who was committed to patient care.

- **Justice versus Mercy**—He'd lost the trust of his colleagues by stepping across an implicit line that says "do not publicly criticize other clinicians." For this, the majority of the partners in the group thought he "deserved" justice—to be punished by being dismissed. The merciful approach would be to give him at least one more chance to change, on the assumption that he would now understand how important his behavior was to his partners.

It took several years of effort, and much angst on his and everyone else's part, but we helped him know what behaviors were unacceptable, reinforced his progress frequently, and supported him when he personally struggled. I don't know if his personality changed, but his behavior did. What we gained was a great colleague, good friend, and valuable clinician for years to come.

Sometimes following your principles, even if you have decision-making skills and experience, can't give you an outcome that everyone feels good about. Here's a story that shows what can happen when people play by different principles. As you read, think about how you would handle the situation, and what principles you would want to stand by.

We were a large, multispecialty medical practice. Pediatrics, family medicine, internists, and obstetricians (ob-gyns). We had been owned and operated by a large health system. As was common during that particular time in the history of the "business of health care," we had recently, in corporate parlance, been "divested." That meant set off to succeed or fail on our own. It was a time of intense competition in the health insurance world, of pressure to make profit margins, of questioning the wisdom of investing in employing clinicians and owning medical practices. I was the medical director of this spun-off, newly independent, medical group, which meant I was the chief executive of the practice and reported to an owner-physician board.

It was important to have ob-gyns in our practice and there were six of them. Our pediatricians liked having new babies come into the practice. It's also thought that women are often the ones who make the health care decisions for their families, so the other primary care clinicians wanted a good ob-gyn group to bring those women into the larger practice.

One of the ob-gyn docs—let's call him Rob—came to me to say he needed to take three months off. He said his mother had dementia, and he and his siblings were taking turns being caregivers. His turn was coming up. Our group, seeing itself as enlightened and progressive, had set up a paid leave policy. So, after consultation with the other ob-gyn clinicians, and a vote by our board members, we told Rob he could have the paid time off. It meant more office time and call for other clinicians, the expense of contracting for additional call coverage, and paying some salary to Rob, but it was deemed important for his well-being and was a "good cause."

A few weeks later, a patient-friend called me with some information. She was in an accelerated teacher training program run by our state. Due to bad economic times and also a teacher shortage, the state was running three-month training sessions. She was surprised to see her ob-gyn physician,

Rob, in the program. Obviously, I was surprised, too, and angry, and fill in any feeling you might feel in this situation and I was likely feeling it too.

I called Rob and asked how things were going. He told me his mom was okay. Then I told him I had heard he was in a teacher training program. He denied it at first, but then admitted it. He said his mom was doing well enough that she didn't need his care, so he decided to use his paid time off to enroll in a program, coincidentally three months in length. He was considering leaving health care at some point and was thinking of teaching as an option (though he ultimately realized during his training program that he missed patient care).

No one in the group was happy—his fellow ob-gyn clinicians, the other primary care colleagues, the board, likely not Rob's displaced patients, either. Rob was a smart, hardworking clinician, and also had a history of being prickly, but this was bad. Really bad. Taking money from the group, leaving his patients, having others work extra to cover for him, being deceptive.

I had the expected emotional response, and it was probably even rational. Even applying Kidder's paradigm wouldn't save Rob from dismissal from the group. He was untruthful and showed no loyalty to the practice. He was acting in his individual interest and not that of the community. How could we continue working with him over the long term? Could there be any mercy in the pursuit of justice?

However, Rob was not dismissed and continued working for the group. Eventually, he became a faculty member at the regional medical school and health system. How could that be? He blamed the group for what he'd done—he was working too hard and was questioning his future as a physician. It was our fault for creating a generous leave policy and not verifying his story. The other ob-gyn clinicians preferred having him back rather than take the chance of not being able to find a replacement. The board voted to keep him. It didn't want to take the chance of a "food fight" with Rob going public. I was stuck trying to be both ethical and pragmatic with someone playing by a different set of rules.

This episode was a reminder that it's not always possible to lead with principles and have everything work out well. But at least to me, it's important to try anyway, if only to avoid becoming a full-time cynic.

CAN YOU PUT YOUR EGO ON THE SHELF?

Becoming a physician is a long process: generally four years of college, four years of medical school, and at least three years of specialty training. It does require a degree of ego strength to get through it. And although the medical professional as a whole is not always held in as high esteem as when Drs. Kildare and Welby practiced on television, individual clinicians are most often still revered (or at least respected) by their patients (and by their own grandparents!). So those already strong egos are frequently reinforced. It's easy to be put on a pedestal, and it can be hard to acknowledge when we're wrong or maybe just don't know something. I've had a number of discussions about whether it's best to tell a patient that I don't know something and need to look it up, or whether I should just leave the exam room under some pretense and come back after checking for the answer on my computer.

> # There are fine lines along the scale from confidence, to over-confidence, to hubris, to arrogance.

Thinking that you're great can help when you need the confidence to deal with tough situations, but it can be dysfunctional when you need to work in a team or need the support of others. There are fine lines along the scale from confidence, to over-confidence, to hubris, to arrogance.

Lao Tzu, the ancient Chinese philosopher wrote, "A leader is best when people barely know he exists. When his work is done, his aim fulfilled, they will all say: We did it ourselves."[8] That often is not how a physician leader wants to see herself or himself. But it is important, at least some of the time, to help your team function to its full potential and to relieve the leader from shouldering every decision and burden.

DO YOU HAVE HUMILITY, AND ARE YOU WILLING AND ABLE TO LEARN?

"Do you wish to rise? Begin by descending. You plan a tower that will pierce the clouds? Lay first the foundation of humility." This saying is attributed to Saint Augustine, and is one of many over the centuries that point us in the same direction. Humility, this human and important trait, is sometimes falsely attributed to weakness. But more and more research has shown that not only are humble people less likely to be polarizing and antagonizing, and less likely to be aggressive and judgmental, they are more likely to have strong beliefs and confidence in their abilities.[9] Having humility can be critical to forming healthy relationships, to being patient with others, and to being able to forgive oneself.[10]

Besides being an important personality trait when it comes to fitting in and in dealing with people, humility is important to learning. In 1969, the management consultant Martin Broadwell described the learning process as:

- Not knowing what you don't know (unconscious incompetence);

- Knowing what you don't know (conscious incompetence);

- Knowing, but needing to think about things (conscious competence); and,

- Doing the right thing without much thought (unconscious competence).[11]

Humility allows someone to admit to themselves they don't know what they don't know and to act to correct that shortcoming. Maybe the most common example, often the subject of humor about the stereotypical male, is the refusal to ask for directions—the idea that we might be diminished by admitting we don't know something. In the health care world, this can be downright dangerous.

As a fourth-year medical student, a nurse asked me to perform a procedure I'd seen performed but had never done myself on a patient. Instead of admitting that and calling for more experienced backup, I went ahead. This was the "see one, do one, teach one" culture common in medical education then. Things quickly went wrong, and we were saved when my mentor happened by. I put the patient at risk, and I was diminished in the eyes of those whose trust I needed.

DO YOU KNOW HOW TO DELEGATE? BEING PART OF A TEAM

Medical training creates, or reinforces, strong-willed people. As we've discussed, such people are often highly competent in their field, adept at decision-making, and confident in their abilities.

But as the breadth of managerial responsibility expands, the ability of any one person to do all that is needed, in a timely fashion, begins to be tested. This is especially true if the manager is trying to practice medicine at the same time. But how do you delegate? As in, get others involved, entrust them with meaningful responsibilities, and not second-guess them or require them to constantly ask permission before acting?

Physicians are detail oriented, and a good manager ensures that details are being taken care of. But he/she may not be able to, or it can be ill-advised to, manage all details by himself or herself. Delegation requires being able to choose good teammates, creating a common vision and goals, being able to let go of the work, but remaining accountable for the outcomes, both good and bad. It means giving meaningful direction, advice, and feedback. A quote from Jim Yong Kim, the recent president of the World Bank, gets right to the heart of this. Dr. Kim is a physician and has a doctorate in anthropology, but he's not an economist. When asked how he navigated his role in international finances and development, he said, "I learned to keep my mouth shut and listen and to let my team make the decisions, unless they reached an impasse, at which point, I needed to decide."[12]

"Teamwork" may seem to be an over-worked management concept. And someone might question why a leader needs to be part of a team. But teamwork is a natural partner with delegation and negotiation skills. Being part of a team assumes you need others and you value what they bring to the table. This point is worth emphasizing: Complementary skills and personalities can be synergistic, as long as the team or the leader can manage conflicts that might arise and continues to value those differences in a way that allows for creativity and collaboration.

Close your eyes and think about your favorite team— maybe one you were part of as an athlete or as a clinician, or think of a sports team you rooted for or admired. As Robert Keidel points out in *Game Plans*,[13] our background and experiences strongly influence our idea of what makes a good team and how we function as team members or leaders.

Prior to Title IX, women mostly were not part of athletic teams, and, if they were, they were individual members of a group effort—e.g., swimming or tennis. More recently, it is more likely than ever that a woman has been on a soccer, lacrosse, field hockey, volleyball, or basketball team. What does a team look like now to a woman? A highly interactive, interdependent group, in which the success of one is hard to separate from that of the whole.

What about men in management? What have their "team" role models been? Are they the stars or the facilitators, are they the quarterbacks or the linemen? The baseball team is, for most of the time, a number of individuals each performing their jobs. Some are stars, some role players, but on the field, other than the pitcher and the catcher and the rare double-play combination, they are standing alone. Football is highly organized, each player having his/her assignment during any specific play. In the past, the quarterback was the orchestrator, calling the plays and giving feedback in the huddle. Now almost every play, on both defense and offense, is radioed in from the coaches on the sidelines. Despite this change, we still think of the quarterback as the top dog, the person who leads by example through his intelligence, work ethic, and skill. He's the one with the direct line to the coaches. He's to be protected at all costs. He's the captain of the ship.

So, with your eyes still closed, what type of team were you seeing (and who was the sports figure you first thought of)? A baseball team of individual stars each doing his/her own thing, interacting at times on the field? A football team with the quarterback telling others what they need to do (and with little discussion or disagreement)? Or a basketball team (say the 1970s Knicks or the Larry Bird Celtics) or a soccer team for which even the stars are dependent upon others to do the work, across the court or field, to give them the ball at the right time and right place, when they're in the right position to make the shot?

Now think about what type of team works best in the emergency department, operating room, or even the medical office. Is it a team in which the leader gives orders, is not inclusive, and doesn't listen or explain? No, it is a team in which success requires each member to understand the goal, the play, his/her role, and to modify his/her behavior based upon the changing needs of the moment and of the health care world. It is a team in which each member is the eyes and ears to the world and is often the face of the team. (The frontline receptionist or medical assistant is often the person who is the first contact, and the representative of the team to the patients.)

My point is that we can't just *tell* people to work as a team. There are too many interpretations of what that means, influenced by prior experiences, role models, and even by different gender roles growing up, to assume there is a common understanding of what a "team" and being a good "team member" is.

The training of a physician is more likely to make him— so often in the past males had the dominant roles on teams— think of himself as the star player. What we want is training that encourages physicians to be the point guards of the basketball team or the setters of the volleyball team: getting the rest of the team involved, being sure they know their roles and the plan.

We can't just tell people to work as a team.

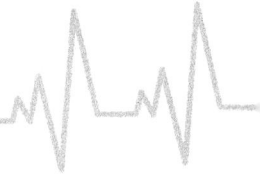

Yes, there are times when the leader needs to take charge, maybe becoming the doer rather than the delegator and facilitator. If the proverbial ship is sinking, in either a patient or a management crisis, then it may be so. But if this is how work is regularly organized, then it's a self-fulfilling prophecy. The staff are reluctant to take responsibility and the manager or leader often feels he/she *has* to do it.

As an organization becomes larger and more complex, it becomes harder for any one person to get things done alone. Remembering Lao Tzu, the leader is someone of whom an outside observer might ask, "What did he do?" Going back to the initial premise of a leader as someone helping others succeed: that person should be giving others the tools, the knowledge, and the authority to do what's needed.

DO YOU HAVE THE ABILITY AND DESIRE TO TEACH?

The word "doctor" in Greek means "teacher." We are expected to help others understand and to share our knowledge. The skeptic reading this may wonder how far away we've strayed from that expectation. If we share our knowledge and our experience, we help others, whether patients or staff, to be better able to participate in decisions, understand why things are happening, care for themselves, and act on their own. That can also relieve some of the burdens we take upon ourselves as clinicians or leaders and managers. Going back to an earlier comment: why did I give that article, "Why Physician Managers Fail," to my colleagues and team? It wasn't only to help them get better; it was also to help myself by encouraging the team to be open with their feedback to me and also to develop their own skills so they could take on more responsibility.

Another reason to be a teacher, to spend time developing staff, is long-term leadership in the form of succession planning. From your first day in a new role, you need to start preparing yourself and your organization for your departure. This is not totally altruistic. I've seen people struggle to leave their jobs or roles because they or their organization didn't have a viable succession plan. This included delays in moving "up the ladder" as there was no one to take over their work.

Another reason to help others be ready to take your place is the value to your organization. Presumably you have loyalty to the mission of your employer, and to your colleagues, and to those whom you serve. Embracing your teaching role increases the likelihood that what you've helped build will be sustained after you're gone.

CAN YOU DEAL WITH PEOPLE? COMMUNICATION, EMPATHY, AND COMPASSION

We can probably accept the idea that listening is a big part of communication.[14] I recently saw one of those signboards that have become commonplace outside churches. The ones with witty and inspirational sayings (there must be a website for these—sometimes I see the same saying at more than one church). This one said, "It's better to be quiet and listen— you already know what you're going to say." Or as more elegantly put by the Dalai Lama: "When you talk, you are only repeating what you already know. But if you listen, you may learn something new."

Being able to sit and listen is extremely important for a clinician. The patient's story can tell us so much about what their problems and concerns are, what they're worried about. Studies have shown that the majority of diagnoses can be made just from the patient's history. Despite knowing this, listening in a meaningful way seems to be hard for many clinicians. Other studies show that most patients are interrupted by the clinician within the first twenty seconds while telling their story![15] In another study of orthopedic physicians, 75 percent of them reported they communicated satisfactorily with their patients. But only 21 percent of those patients believed they had had satisfactory communication. Why the impatience on the part of the physicians, and why the disparity in perceptions? My guess is that we're trained to make quick judgments, to move instantaneously from diagnosis to doing something about a problem, and we are under intense time pressure. There is always another patient to be seen. Successful managers must break any predilection for jumping out of their seats and declaring they know what to do. If she/he is not a good listener, this skill will need to be learned.[16]

Being able to sit and listen is extremely important for a clinician.

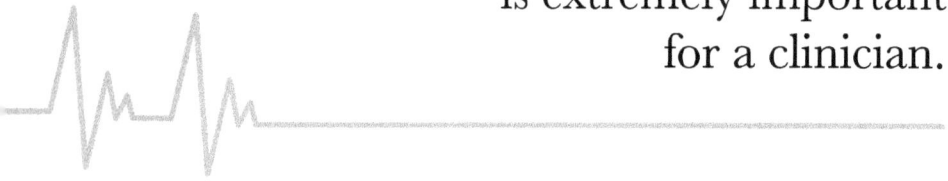

Listening, especially being an active listener, validates the importance of the person speaking. What is an active listener? Someone who is attentive to the speaker (e.g., not staring at a cell phone or laptop screen), someone who nods or verbally acknowledges what they are hearing, and, especially, someone who asks clarifying and follow-up questions.

Another good reason to listen first, and speak (or act) later is so you don't say or do something rash that you may later regret. Give yourself a chance to consider what to do, including getting more information. More than once I've regretted speaking before my mind had a chance to be smart. I've chastened a patient for being late to an appointment before knowing they were unavoidably tied up (at a funeral, by a traffic accident).

I've also allowed my rush to judgment to lead to a few managerial errors. A manager on our team once came to me to complain about a decision that another manager had made. It seemed in contradiction to what I'd laid out as a plan. I called in the supposed culprit and in a not-too-friendly tone of voice told her I was disappointed. She then told me that my boss had instructed her to do what she had done. She assumed I knew about it. Only then did I realize I had not done my job of communicating and managing "up" to other leaders. I'd made two mistakes: the first was not to have done all the legwork for an important decision. The second was to accuse a good manager of something before I had done enough listening.

If you haven't invested the time into listening, it's also particularly hard to be empathetic. Not only patients, but your team and staff need to know you're willing to take the time to hear them out, that you understand and care about what they are feeling and have to say. Otherwise, you may be just another impersonal cog in the machine of health care for patients.

We discussed earlier the idea of "putting your ego on the shelf." In the context of communication that leads to the question of how much to share your own feelings, shortcomings, and fears with a patient or with colleagues. I've read pros and cons of doing so. Sharing with an asthmatic patient that you have asthma too, how it impacts your life, and how particular treatments work and help can be powerfully empathetic. As a manager, being able to say to a team member, "That way you were treated by Dr. X must have made you feel awful—when I was criticized by my boss I felt that way," can be a good approach if you are sincere (but don't make it all about yourself). I was surprised that several years after sharing with a colleague my story about losing my management position, he reminded me of it. It had an impact on him; he felt he could trust me enough to tell me about his own management struggles since I'd had similar challenges.

A particular quality for which clinicians are trained—being objective, calm, even stoic, and neutral in tone—can be detrimental both clinically and managerially if it comes across as lacking empathy and compassion. There is a scene in the movie *All That Jazz* in which Roy Schneider, playing a fictionalized Bob Fosse, stands in front of a mirror after waking in the morning, pries his eyes open, puts in his contact lenses, and says, "It's showtime, folks." The leader is always on stage—she can't be faking it. She needs to be engaged, energetic, passionate, and to be sure her heart is in the part. She needs to be cognizant of how others see her. It is always "show time." The door needs to be "open" for listening and being willing to help.

CAN YOU SET AND AGREE ON PRIORITIES?

There's a line in an old sixties song by the Youngbloods, "A dreamer's dream can only be reality if two dreamers dream." For a leader, that translates into this truism: To get something important done means that someone else needs to consider it important too.

Underlying this truth is the management reality that the higher one gets in an organization, the more help she/he needs to be effective. This reflects the importance of humility—knowing you can't do it alone and bringing into play all your skills in forming and empowering a team.

How does this work in practical application? For one, your staff and other stakeholders in the organization need to understand the general environment, as well as the particular issue being worked on. This will require as many meetings and as much time providing background information as necessary. Does the lowest level employee need as much prep work as the direct reports? It depends.

Here's a real-life example: the incorporation of nurse practitioners into a primary care practice. Years ago, folks at a large, integrated health system realized that only 30–40 percent of their patients were accepting offered appointments with nurse practitioners as alternatives to physician appointments.[17] As this was explored, one issue that turned up was an inadequate effort to explain to patients just what a nurse practitioner was and could do—the training, skills, their expertise in particular areas, their ability to order tests, to write prescriptions, and their ready access to physician backup when desired or needed. Physicians had not been explaining to patients that nurse practitioners were part of their team. The health system had not provided informational materials to their population of patients. They also found that the frontline office staff were at least an equal part of the knowledge gap. They did not know, or could not articulate, the things that the team wanted the patients to know. They are "nurses"—*but nurses can't order tests and medications, can they? What kinds of problems can they deal with? Will I need to come back again to see the "real" doctor?* Once the practice spent time working with the receptionists, clerks, and assistants, acceptance of appointments with nurse practitioners went up to 70–80 percent with appropriate patients.

This experience was a good example of how a focused goal increases engagement of the staff and the success of the implementation. In my experience, and borne out by management studies, people can only deal with a few management priorities at any one time (this also applies to multitasking, which it's now been shown is not a particularly good way of doing work). I generally use the rule of three. If my priorities don't rank in your top three, it's not very likely you'll spend time and energy helping me accomplish my goals. So I will need to help you understand why my goal is important and why your help is needed. Maybe I need to help you clear your agenda, or I need to adjust my timeline to be more realistic.

Here's an example: I wanted to change the team structure in a large primary care office, and we had worked out all the reasons this was good for patient care and eventually would make life easier for the clinicians. But the frontline manager pushed back that the clinicians were unhappy—not necessarily with the new ideas, but with their ability to cope with the changes at the moment. It was a time of year when there was a lot of illness in the community, the staff were in the middle of a change in the mechanics of the electronic medical record, and a long-time colleague had just retired. Any other significant change at this time would overload them and might not be successful. It's been attributed to Che Guevara that "you can't talk philosophy to people when they're starving." The practice was not literally starving, but they were stretched to their work limits. I was convinced to hold off for several months until the current issues could be resolved and then to try again. Seeing my empathy and willingness to shift priorities to include their well-being, the clinicians saw they had some control over the process and of their daily lives and were then able to partner fully in the desired change.

The leader also needs to do an assessment (some call this a "force-field analysis") of what barriers there might be that are preventing others from helping out. Are the staff afraid (thinking the new plan may eliminate or negatively change their job), not willing to admit they don't know something (don't assume they understand the new idea or technology as well as you do), or have been given different goals and direction by another manager? This last possibility is particularly important in a highly matrixed organization. In one organization I worked for, I was responsible for all practice operations, but there were chiefs of internal medicine and family medicine who had academic oversight of "my" clinicians. There were times when something I wanted to do caused a clinician to complain to their chief. I learned that I should work with the chiefs to get ourselves on the same page before trying to implement changes.

We'll get more into change management in the second part of this book. For now, it's important to note that the leader/manager needs to have enough understanding and empathy, and enough ability to defer her/his own goals, to be sure the team and staff are ready to be full collaborators.

CAN YOU NEGOTIATE? ACCEPTING THAT THERE MIGHT BE MORE THAN ONE RIGHT ANSWER

Negotiation is a way for people who might have different goals, and paths to those goals, to realize the commonality of those goals. At that point, negotiation can then help them bridge the remaining gaps so they can each

I learned that I should work with the chiefs to get ourselves on the same page before trying to implement changes.

achieve as much of what they want as possible and maybe even things they hadn't known they wanted.

Clinicians, especially physicians, traditionally are not trained to be flexible in their goals and behavior, to search for a middle ground. We clinicians very often think of ourselves as scientists. We don't spend nearly as much time learning "the art of medicine" as we do the best or right way of diagnosing and treating patients. We have to make the "right" decisions because we may not have a second chance. The "there's one right answer, and I know it" maxim is reinforced by the tenets of evidence-based medicine—the idea that decisions should be based upon what has been proven by scientific studies to work. All our education makes it hard to accept that others might have other, equally good, ways of doing something. It is somewhat paradoxical since, for most medical conditions, there is more than one diagnostic approach and more than one therapeutic option. An example is the treatment of high blood pressure. There are at least sixty medications available for this, as well as a few treatments not using drugs. As clinicians, we need to accept that there is not one perfect way of treating high blood pressure.

As leaders and managers, we need to accept that there is most often not one perfect approach to doing that job either. When we live in a "take it or leave it," zero-sum game world, we not only deprive ourselves of other good ideas and ways of increasing value, but we increase the likelihood of resistance to our ideas and initiatives. In physics, there is the principle that every action has an equal and opposite reaction. Human

> ## As clinicians, we need to accept that there is not one perfect way.

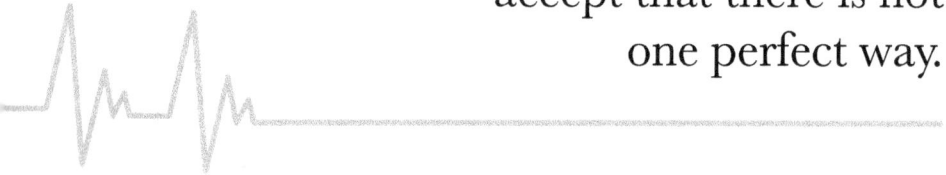

behavior frequently mirrors that phenomenon. At one time, our health system brought in a physician leader from another organization. When I first met with him, he told me that if he had his way, he'd get rid of every physician working in our practice. That statement probably had the shock value he wanted. Nobody wanted to be seen as being in opposition to any of the ideas he proposed. But soon our lack of enthusiasm, and our fear of doing something he might not like, made making any changes, even if wise, impossible. He had cut off the possibility that a give-and-take, a challenging of ideas, might be a way of increasing value for all concerned.

Eventually, he had to bring in another physician leader, one with empathy and listening skills, to be his go-between with the rest of us. Only then did he get the necessary buy-in and energy from us to make things work better.

Remember my earlier statement: "Nobody ever died because of a management decision"? This may not be totally true. You can imagine a decision to hire a doctor who turns out not to have adequate skills and puts patients at risk; or a decision that negatively impacts access to care, such as changing the way patients can contact a practice, unintentionally making it harder for patients to get in touch in an emergency. But hopefully you get the gist. That is, rarely are management decisions life or death, rarely do they need to be made in the moment without adequate due diligence, and rarely is there only one way of doing something—there may often be completely viable, alternative approaches.

Being able to accept and to negotiate differences has multiple values. Most obviously, someone else might have a better idea. Maybe they are closer to the problem and can see why something might or might not work more clearly than you can from your executive desk. Maybe they think differently or don't have the same biases as you. Or maybe they have developed a better problem-solving approach. There is a system of creativity called "lateral thinking," first described by Edward de Bono in 1967, which is the subject of several of his books in which he gives insight on how to train your mind to think more creatively.[18] Lateral thinking is similar to the approach of imagining a future and then working backward to understand how to get there. Both ways of developing ideas can allow us to address problems by imagining solutions and original answers, which cannot be arrived at via deductive or logical means. At the very least, at times of change, an organization can benefit from this approach when traditional solutions are unlikely to get the desired result. A leader who comes into a change or decision process thinking they already have the right answer will find it hard to give space to other, maybe better, ideas.

Another reason to encourage, not discourage, others to be "right" is to empower them to tell you when you yourself are off path and could do better. I once worked for an executive who told us, "I need you to disagree with me. I pay you to disagree with me." He often prefaced his comments by saying, "This may need to be added to my book of stupid ideas." His management meetings were sometimes raucous. But we were always encouraged to participate. We were empowered to come up with ideas, and we knew they would be challenged without personal attacks or permanent consequences. These unruly sessions were a type of negotiation, ending with better plans than those with which we had entered the room. I also worked for a leader who didn't want to be disagreed with. That resulted in managers competing with one another to show how much they approved of the leader's ideas.

Encouraging dissent and being willing to negotiate takes ego strength and humility. Being successful is highly

Encouraging dissent and being willing to negotiate takes ego strength and humility.

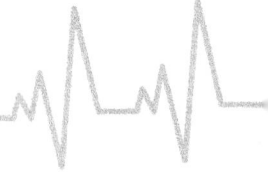

dependent upon having established mutual goals, mores, and respect. It requires the leader to be explicit and consistent in his/her expectations. This means being able to admit mistakes, and not blaming others when things go wrong. This applies to management problems, as well as clinical ones. Too often a clinician will blame a colleague when there is a poor outcome, or, even worse, blame the patient. This behavior can carry over to management problems—the proverbial "throwing under the bus" of a team or staff member. It's important to know that such behavior is usually transparent to other managers, and probably to your staff too. It adds to the reluctance of others to take risks, to make decisions, to disagree when appropriate, or to be willing to help you, for fear of private or public shaming.

Not only do physician managers need to ask themselves if they are good at negotiating, they need to ask if they are able to be negotiated *with*.

CAN YOU LET GO OF NEEDING TO WIN?

A close relative of the difficulty all humans have of wanting to be right is the competitive urge to win, to own all the "marbles." Clinicians are not immune to this desire. If anything, they are honed by medical training, and by the perceived and real embarrassment of making clinical mistakes, to be supercompetitive. The fear of young physicians of being grilled and embarrassed on morning hospital rounds is real, and the need to survive stressful challenges becomes internalized. When that young physician later becomes a leader or manager, this can carry over into refusing to compromise, and, worse, by undermining others in word and/or deed. It can also show up in creating enemies—us versus them. It's not uncommon for clinicians and clinician managers to bad-mouth and blame non-clinician managers, medical records personnel, information technology staff, or other clinical departments. In some instances, there will be tension between emergency department staff and the inpatient team, or between the inpatient team and the outpatient services.

Our hospital had one of the busiest emergency departments in the country. Patients regularly had long waits to get care due to how many people needed to be seen. There was constant bickering between the emergency department team and the inpatient team about who was to blame. Was it the former for being slow in evaluating patients, or the latter for being slow in discharging inpatients and preparing beds for patients needing to be admitted from the emergency department? Only when the emergency department and the inpatient service were able to agree that if anyone would be a winner in this disagreement it would certainly not be the patients, did they stop blaming and start working together. With the needs of the patients in focus, they were then able to agree upon viable solutions.

It takes a good soul to maintain the approach that criticisms and concerns are dealt with privately, that scapegoating doesn't solve problems, and that there is limited value in creating a bunker, us-versus-them mentality.

Speaking of needing to win, all too often leaders and managers find themselves fighting the wrong battles. It's understandable that a health care clinician cannot ignore details regarding patients. That mildly abnormal laboratory test needs to be repeated to be sure it doesn't mean anything. That questionable spot on an x-ray might be an early cancer. But a leader or manager needs to come to grips with not fighting over every detail. It's too exhausting and time-consuming. I knew a non-clinician executive who felt he'd been wronged by a physician manager. At every opportunity he tried to undermine the physician. But the physician was well respected and had made many friends during his years in the organization. It was a battle the executive could never win, and he shouldn't have fought it. It only made him look petty, and he used up whatever political capital he'd had on a useless fight.

CAN YOU SAY NO?

While many physicians have strong egos and often have the need to maintain control, to fight every battle and win every argument, when it comes to unpleasant conversations, they often behave just the opposite. Many want to avoid conflict, to not disappoint others, to be "likeable" in their professional and personal lives.

In patient care, this can be seen as not wanting to give bad news to patients or by communicating that news in a vague manner that allows different interpretations. An example is the avoidance of the use of the word "cancer," instead saying there's a "spot" or "growth." After all, the clinician is trained to believe, and there are many experiences that confirm, that there is often at least some hope in seemingly dire circumstances.

In management, the desire not to face up to a bad situation or an aversion to bear ill tidings can result in delays in making decisions. An example is when someone agonizes over whether a situation, such as employee performance, is remediable or not.

A mentor once told me that it often takes more energy and angst to delay taking action than any potential benefit of delaying an unpleasant decision. In a "fish or cut bait" choice, is it really worth the effort to delay? Is it maybe a better idea to decide and move forward? In practical terms: Is a business practice or an employee's performance worth the effort to try to improve it? What is the opportunity cost to not just moving on?

Here's an example: Our primary care group had a physician who was well liked by her peers. She was sociable, having colleagues to her home for dinner parties. She was caring, always asking about the well-being of our families. She was collegial, never saying no if you needed someone to cover your night on-call. Her office was a bit disorganized; her patient medical recordkeeping could be short on details, but these were initially viewed as just being eccentricities, which she could eventually fix. Shortly thereafter, though, a few clinicians mentioned to the practice manager that they were no longer sure of some of her medical decision-making. While covering for another clinician, she might see a patient and change a bunch of medications. She might encourage the use of vitamins or nutritional supplements when it seemed more traditional treatments were in order. Yet no one wanted to discuss these issues with her, nor did they want management to do so. Nobody wanted to hurt her feelings; nobody wanted to lose a friendly and helpful colleague.

The management team then heard that some of her colleagues didn't want her seeing their patients when they themselves were not available. Their trust in her judgment had eroded even more. This scenario played out over at least six months (you may be wondering why management didn't know what was going on and had not been more proactive—indeed, this was a symptom of a lack of trust in management, and soon after led to a change). And still nobody wanted to talk with her. Eventually, I was asked in my role in quality assurance to investigate, to propose a plan, and to do something about the problem.

After talking with all the peers and reviewing patient records, I saw there was objective information, as well as sentiment, that showed we had a choice to make. Should we choose a lot of mentoring and monitoring, with no guarantee we would see her improve or that other clinicians would be reassured? Or should we find a graceful way for her to leave the practice? With great trepidation, and more delay, I arranged to speak with her. I told her what we were concerned about. She seemed annoyed and asked who "we" were. She asked what evidence I had. I explained that I'd spoken with all the other clinicians and the consensus was they were uncomfortable with her practice style and decision-making, but they'd been afraid to hurt her feelings.

I thought she would become angry, or at least cry (I was about to myself). Instead, she said she was relieved. She'd been unhappy with work for a long time, but didn't want to let her colleagues and friends down. Knowing they didn't want her there, and they cared for her as a person, allowed her to leave without anger or remorse. She went on to work in an urgent care center—it was better for her schedule and family needs, and there weren't as many complex patients. Over the subsequent years, she remained in that practice as a well-respected clinician.

Nobody wanted to deliver bad news to her or to make an uncomfortable decision. The result was an extended period of unhappiness. We could have tried to work with her to improve her decision-making or her organizational skills, but by not facing up to the situation earlier, we missed that opportunity. By eventually taking an honest approach, we were able to do something that took into account both her and our needs. This, in essence, required being able to say "no" to her, thereby taking the risk of causing her to be angry and upset and having to bear that guilt myself

Thinking back to the decision-making paradigm of truth versus loyalty, there does come a time, especially when patient well-being is jeopardized, when the need to honestly deal with a situation is greater than the desire to help a friend. And in this, as in many other instances (though not all!), can actually be the more friendly, meaningful path to take.

ARE YOU SURROUNDING YOURSELF WITH PEOPLE JUST LIKE YOU?

A corollary to the last example of wanting others to like us is the tendency to choose people we like as coworkers—people who make us feel good when we see them or who are just like us—even if they may not be the best fit for the job. Once again, this is not solely a characteristic of clinician leaders.

There will be more detail on selecting staff and teammates in the second section of this book.

I've observed several health systems in which the clinical leaders are mostly from internal medicine. In one system, this then switched to family medicine, before drifting to the surgical specialties. Not uncommonly in health systems, the newly chosen leader brings in parts of his/her team from his/her previous role. Familiarity can certainly help with continuity, but it may result in a reluctance of team members to disagree and a reluctance of "outsiders" to challenge or critique. It then requires an active effort to seek diverse opinions and create dialogue instead of that being the default way of behaving. It also can lead to strategic and tactical decisions that are weighted toward the needs and worldview of that particular type of clinician—or maybe just creating the suspicion that it does.

It is now recognized that it is important to the outcomes and morale of an organization to have a diversity of backgrounds, interests, and experience on the team.[19] Soon after I joined one health system as an executive, I mentioned to the chief executive officer that all but three of his twenty-person senior team were White men, and most of them were grey haired, if they had hair at all. He said he realized this was a problem and was trying to figure out how to change it. It is usually easier to have a proactive diversity strategy in place rather than to try to change a preexisting management structure after the fact. A related issue is favoring people who have the same interests or affinities—come from the same geography, have the same hobbies, look like us, and use that as subconscious (or even conscious) reasons to make personnel decisions. You may enjoy talking with someone who shares your interests in gardening or travel, or who went to school where you went, but that is usually not a good reason to hire them.

It is fair to question whether I'm just suggesting a different type of prejudice, a counter-snobbism for its own sake. But the health care literature contains ample—and an increasing number of—studies on the real and perceived barriers to care when clinicians and management teams become internally focused or don't adequately reflect and represent the communities they serve. A few examples include inadequate responses to chest pain in women in emergency rooms, inadequate pain relief provided to Hispanics, inner city hospitals with non-minority management teams being perceived as non welcoming to the needs of the community, and Black patients feeling they are not listened to by White health care professionals.

THE COST OF FAILURE; THE PRICE OF SUCCESS

There are costs incurred if a manager or leader does not perform well, whether she/he is a clinician or otherwise. The costs are to the individual who has struggled, to the community, and to the organization. The obvious problems include the consequences of poor decisions and wasted efforts. Putting a manager in place often takes an expensive recruiting process, on-the-job training, and a period of time for her/him to become fully productive. For clinicians who may not have had insight into the difficulty of management and the personal commitments it requires, it may be a significant blow to their self-image and feeling of self-worth. For people who have rarely "failed" personally or professionally, it can be particularly hurtful.

Not wanting to admit failure, they may try to hang on or delay seeking help for too long, damaging their relationships and impeding the work of the organization. If they have been chosen for the "wrong" reasons—such as their popularity as clinicians or their friendships—other senior executives may be reluctant to speak up about their performance.

It is not rare that a failed clinician manager is then lost to the community. She/he may feel it was not her/his fault (many people would first blame others before admitting their own need to improve) and become embittered. The result is someone who decides to leave her/his practice, patients, and colleagues to start afresh. Rarely have I seen the result instead being a plan for personal and organizational investment in improvement.

On the other hand, there is a price to success. That is, we need to invest in the hiring and performance of our leaders and managers. This investment should clearly include the process to select candidates in a systematic fashion,

There is a price to success.

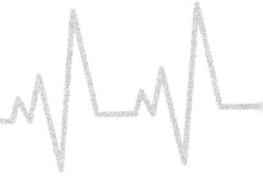

with specific, pre-considered criteria that include the need to have a balanced, collaborative team. It also means both the clinician and the system need to invest in educational and training opportunities that develop management and leadership skills. This may mean time off-site to learn from outside experts or from peers from other organizations. Or it may mean having an internal program for management development. It also should include resources for proactive mentorship and for interventions and problem-solving (and for an honest evaluation and feedback process, so poor performance is not allowed to drag on). The price is therefore not just money, but time, detailed work on developing a culture and philosophy of leadership, and soul-searching.

Here's a recent quote from Nick Green, the CEO of Thrive Market, that nicely summarizes some of the points I've made so far:

> People probably overemphasize the importance of decisiveness and action. Both are very important as a leader. But I think, very often, just as important is listening and seeking perspectives. I've had a number of humbling mistakes that I've made, most of which were because I moved too fast and thought I had the answer. And I've

been consistently amazed when I go into the organization to get feedback, how insightful and how much knowledge and understanding and perspective there is when you listen to your people.[20]

WHY PHYSICIAN/CLINICIAN MANAGERS FAIL AND HOW THEY CAN SUCCEED TAKEAWAYS

- Start with acknowledging that good clinicians don't necessarily make good managers; it can't be assumed that being a good and well-liked clinician is enough to be a good manager or leader.

- Some of the personal attributes and success factors of clinicians may actually interfere with being successful at management. Embrace the following lessons to create the possibility of success as a leader:

- Commit to a vision.

- Apply principles: truth versus loyalty; the individual versus the community; short-term versus long-term; justice versus mercy.

- Shelve your ego: be willing to give in to others and know what you don't know.

- Have the humility to listen: accept that others might have good, better, or at least helpful ideas.

- Delegate to your team.

- Cultivate the desire and ability to be a teacher.

- Deal with people with communication, empathy, and compassion, remembering that communication should be two-way.

- Set and agree on priorities before taking action.

- Learn to negotiate and tolerate more than one answer.

- Let go of needing to win.

- Learn to say no.

- Surround yourself with diverse and complimentary skillsets, not people who are just like you.

- Failure has implications for the individual, for the organization, and for the health care community;

- The individual and the organization should invest the time and money into management and leadership skill development, as well as into having a structure that supports the individual and the teams.

PART II

Leadership and Management Skills

In Part I, we spoke about some strengths and also about some unfortunate flaws, sometimes critical, for management performance of and by physicians and other clinicians. Though these strengths and weaknesses are not solely characteristic of health care leaders and managers, I've asked you to accept that what a physician or other health care clinician learns or finds helpful in regards to patient care may interfere with her/his success in management and leadership roles.

We can debate whether these characteristics existed before the individual entered into clinical training or were learned during that training and subsequent clinical practice—a nature-versus-nurture, chicken-or-egg question. Years ago, I came across a study that suggested internal medicine physicians more often had Type A personalities than did family physicians, and family physicians were more often Type A than were pediatricians. More recently, there's been a plethora of studies that try to predict which Myers-Briggs types are likely to choose which medical specialty and if the likelihood of success in a particular specialty is related to personality type. [21] There are even online articles trying to tie a person's Harry Potter "house" affinity (altruistic Hufflepuff or devious Slytherin) to their success as a physician! But even if such things are true, it still begs the question if someone with a particular personality type chooses a field in which they inherently feel more comfortable (e.g., where they can be detail oriented, controlling, or thrive on chaos), or if training and work requirements cause them to develop these qualities. [22]

No matter the reason(s), for our purposes, we're interested in understanding if, and how, performance can be improved by learning and improving skills. And my answer is: "definitely yes!"

In an interview with Thomas Friedman, the leadership and ethics consultant Dov Seidman suggested there are four things someone needs to do to be an effective leader. [23] To paraphrase, they are 1) build coalitions; 2) trust people and inspire trust; 3) be caring and compassionate; 4) have humility. Seidman went on to say that great leaders trust people with the truth. The skills we're about to discuss will go a long way to meeting those needs and to helping yourself and others be successful.

FOUR
Skill #1—Humility

I suggest that the first skill for physician managers to nurture is humility. As discussed in Part I, a lack of humility can blind people to understanding that they don't know everything, that they can learn and improve, that they are not alone, and that they don't need to be afraid to ask for advice and help.

Does humility only come from upbringing and inherent personality traits? Is it part of a learned or adopted worldview or way of fitting in? Current research has not determined if humility can be taught to adults. But what is important is that it should not be suppressed, and it is a trait or skill that should be prized. Studies suggest that only 10–15 percent of adults rate highly for humility on psychological testing. [24] These people should be sought-after members of the leadership and management team. By listening, reserving judgment, speaking carefully, and looking for ways to bring others together, they can be the glue, if not the conscience, of a team.[25]

It should be clear that humility is not a sign of weakness. It is not the same as passivity. It can be a way of strongly

Humility is not a sign of weakness.

working toward a goal. It allows us to recognize the strengths and weaknesses in ourselves and in those around us and to convey empathy. Practicing humility requires deep conviction and faith in your own abilities. It means having a strong ego, one that is not afraid of being diminished by seeking advice, and admitting to needing the help of others. Gandhi lived humbly and practiced humility, yet his nonviolent resistance was an active and forceful approach to societal and political change and was galvanizing and courageous.

HUMILITY TAKEAWAYS

- It is not a sign of weakness to accept that no one knows everything, that learning new skills, whether they are interpersonal or technical, needs to be an ongoing effort.

- Humility is an essential leadership strength that needs to be nurtured.

FIVE
Skill #2—Building the Team

"Bad teams, nobody leads. Good teams, coaches lead.
Great teams, everybody leads."[26]
—JOHN BACON, *leadership consultant and high school hockey coach*

Earlier, we talked about the risks that come from choosing staff who are just like us. So how do you make the right choices?

ASKING THE RIGHT QUESTIONS

I suggest first laying out a number of questions, and then working with your current colleagues, staff, and team to refine the list and provide some answers. Here are some potential questions and answers, to give you a place to start:

- What is the position to be filled, and why are you filling it? This may seem obvious, but you may find that not everyone is in agreement. Maybe the current workers feel they can absorb the work themselves, leaving more funds for other uses (or for their own compensation). Maybe the timing isn't right for a recruiting process, or other recent hires haven't had time to be adequately integrated into the team.

- Could a different skill set make a similar or even better contribution to your organization? If the opening is for a clinician, might a nurse practitioner or physician assistant be a better fit? Maybe she/he would provide more of an urgent care skill, or have a personality or interests that complement those of others—is she/he a good listener; good teacher; interested in women's health or diabetes; a calming presence; have leadership potential?

- What's your definition of a "team"? Does it matter if the new hire is a "lone ranger" or does she/he need to fit a role that requires coordination with another, say sharing that person's practice? In management, this might mean looking for someone who can complement the personality and style of someone, including yourself. I was fortunate to choose a non-physician partner who rejoiced in interpersonal relationships and in storytelling. Both those traits/skills were ones which were needed, but which I was not good at. Is the new hire intended to be a teacher, mentor, or evolve into a leader? Or is being "just" a good worker all that's wanted right now? Sometimes the most important need is for someone to come in and reliably do the work every day without complaint.

- Do you have an immediate need or can you wait to hire until the best, or at least a better, candidate comes along? It consumes time and energy to go through a hiring process and can be expensive if you need to enlist a recruiting service. But it also consumes time and energy to have to deal with a bad hire, and is potentially painful for colleagues, staff, and patients. Well-functioning teams depend upon stability, and they want to be able to trust you to take their interests to heart.

- If the candidate is not quite right but has potential, do you have sufficient time and resources for some training and ramp up?

- What about providing a growth opportunity for someone already in the organization? Not only might you have the right person nearby, but the message you send to others can help to retain talent and improve morale.

- Is this hire an opportunity to improve the diversity of the organization (racial, ethnic, gender)? A good way of getting diverse and innovative ideas is to have a diverse workforce and team, not just a lot of people with the same backgrounds, experiences, and perspectives.

- And finally, and very importantly, can you use this hire to raise the level of your team? It might seem hard to define this, but consider that having good people in your organization attracts other good people to want to join you. Remember that manager who told me that if he had his way, he'd fire all the physicians and start over? Well, he didn't fire anyone, but some did leave because of the threat and feeling they were not wanted. The manager then succeeded in hiring five of the best-trained, experienced, and personable clinicians that can be imagined. Those folks, and a few of the leftovers like me, formed a core that continued to attract new recruits and a self-sustaining, high-quality team for the next fifteen years. As I became the manager of that practice, my work was easier because of those five folks who raised the level of our group.

THE SEARCH

By the way, should you use an outside recruiter? That really depends upon whether you have an in-house resource and a ready pool of candidates. You and your management team also need the time, interest, and skill to screen applicants. You also need to assess what you're willing to pay for a search firm. I've found that if you do use a recruiter, it is best not to have them pre-interview or prep candidates. More than once, I've found candidates having prepared answers that initially led me to believe they were better put together and more able than turned out to be the case. You really don't want someone selling a candidate to you, but rather serving up some choices. Hire a recruiter as you might an employee; talk with her/his references and try to decipher if she/he wants to be with you for a quick "hit" or for a longer relationship. If you do use a recruiter, try to establish a mutually beneficial relationship, building an understanding of your needs and trust.

To reinforce what I said earlier, I've found it best to work with the team or practice to help define the need, role, and characteristics of the new hire. If there is not an early agreement, not only can candidates be given mixed messages, but onboarding and acculturation can be impeded. And, yes, staff can accidentally or intentionally torpedo the hiring process. Once I explained in detail to a candidate what opportunities he/she would have for advancement. But I hadn't gone over that with the other interviewers, and they ended up discouraging the candidate because they were not aware that advancement was a possibility.

Importantly, be asking: Is this a good match? That question encompasses much of what is above, but includes more. It takes into account not just what you want and need, but what the candidate wants and needs. She/he might be a great person, with great experience, but if the job is not what the candidate wants or is likely to be good at, then there's a good chance you will both be unhappy.

Here are a couple of real-life experiences. On several occasions, I was recruiting for primary care clinicians and had applicants with great training and personalities but no primary care experience. Both had gone into emergency or urgent care medicine after their training to help earn a good income to pay off their educational debts. Both had wanted, and still wanted, to become primary care clinicians. But both failed in our practice. Why? They had become comfortable and attuned to the so-called "treat and street" mindset of an urgent/emergent care clinician. They knew diabetes and hypertension, but they were stimulated more by dealing with acute illness, rather than by chronic care. They liked people but didn't prioritize establishing long-term relationships. Remember the story about the internist in our group who found happiness in urgent care? We loved these folks as people, we respected their knowledge, but our job was not right for them. They were gone within a year.

Sometimes the mismatch is not really the "fault" of the candidate but is at least partly the fault of your own group (or even beyond). In our primary care group, we once had a resignation when we were already a bit short-staffed due to the rapid growth of our patient population. As a result, all the partners were putting in extra time in the office, as well as taking extra night calls. We found a physician with good training and experience, but I was worried it was not a good match—she had done mostly pulmonary medicine, and a lot of inpatient care, but now said she wanted to be in primary care. She was living in Hawaii, but we were on the East Coast, and she had no family or friends in our part of the world. However, she interviewed well on the phone and we had her come for a visit. Because this needed to be a decision based upon a single visit, we arranged a dinner for her and her husband with our primary care internists and their spouses. After the evening, all the physicians voted to offer her a job, and she soon joined the practice. She was gone within two months. It turned out she no longer wanted to see patients in the hospital (a part of our role), didn't want to share patients (with partners and nurse practitioners), and didn't like the oversight that came with a group practice. These were all, technically, "on her." But in retrospect, she had given hints during the interview process of these preferences. Why did we ignore them? When I went back to the partners to do a "post-mortem," I realized we had downplayed or ignored these concerns. I found that their votes were driven by wanting to fill the open slot in the call schedule. That turned out to be the prime reason most had voted to offer her a job— not that she was a good fit. And some of the physicians cast blame upon their spouses; the call rotation was onerous and the spouses were applying pressure for their partners to be at home more. So we opted to hire someone to fill one shorter-term need, while failing to be concerned that she didn't fit a longer-term need. It would have been better to find another solution for the call rotation because, as a result of the mis-hire, we lost time and money, and damaged morale.

Once you've defined and answered your questions, have a picture of what you think will be the right characteristics of a candidate (including having prioritized needs and wants), and have clarified your recruiting process, next is to have an approach and plan for choosing the right person.

First and foremost, my advice is, "Don't fall in love!" Well, not ever in your life, but not with a candidate. This needs to be a rational, objective process. It should not be one in which you set your heart on someone and forget to check all your boxes. Too often when we fall in love with a candidate, it's because they are like us or have interests that are similar to ours (i.e., education, geographic origin, specialty, hobbies). Finding out someone is a bicyclist, and you are also, and you have a good conversation about that, does not automatically make them a good fit as a clinician or manager.

INTERVIEWING

An interview should help you answer some specific questions. What kind of person is the candidate, how does she/he communicate, what's their experience and skill, and how does that help fill your needs? You'll also want to be sure they know what the job really is, remembering that a poor fit trumps a good *curriculum vitae* (CV). Once you determine that this is someone you might hire, it's a chance to begin selling him/her on, and orienting him/her to, your organization.

That's a lot to accomplish, so it's wise to have a plan. Who will be part of the interview team, who will make a preliminary call, who will do a tour, and who might share a meal? Do you need to have a prepared list of questions for the team with assignments of who will ask what? Are there

My advice is, "Don't fall in love!"

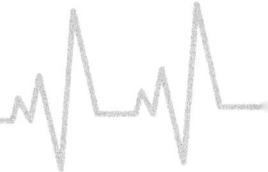

questions that are off-limits? How will you gather the information from the interviewers? When, and by whom, will there be follow-up? Here are suggestions about the interview process informed by my readings and experiences:[27]

- There should be a preliminary phone call before a visit. That saves a lot of wasted time. For example, sometimes it's as simple as finding out the candidate didn't realize what a group practice means, and it's clear she/he is more interested in having complete control over her/his practice structure and daily life. Or she/he might not have realized the call responsibilities. You might hear that she/he doesn't plan on relocating due to a spouse or other needs and she/he was thinking of commuting an hour twice a day. Or she/he is planning on only being in the job for a year or two and then moving on due to further training plans for herself/himself or a spouse. If you have an in-house recruiter, and you trust that person and she/he understands the needs of the position and the culture you're building, then it's okay for that person to do the introductory call.

- You should have a team of folks to meet the candidate. If there will be more than one visit, the team can be spread over those occasions. There should be a list of questions for each team member and the information she/he is meant to impart. Candidates often don't appreciate being asked the same questions by multiple people throughout a long, stressful day. I try to have all the incumbents in a practice site meet with a candidate for that site (should the recruit be for a clinical role) and all the fellow managers and future direct reports (if it is for a management role). What if there has been an incumbent who is leaving? It's easier to put that person on the interview team if she/he has been a good employee and has been happy with her/his job. For example, hearing that someone doesn't want to leave, but has to for family reasons, and really wants to be sure a good person takes her/his place (especially her/his patients, if it's clinical) can be a powerful recruiting tool. The unhappy employee? It depends—if she/he is going voluntarily, it may work to have her/him speak with a candidate; not if it's involuntary. In either case, try to be honest with the candidate about what's going on. It's better she/he hears it from you.

- Yes, there should be a tour, including a visit to the practice site or management office. The person giving the tour can be a recruiter or a manager. There's a lot that can be learned from how the candidate comports herself or himself, how engaged she/he is, and what questions she/he has. When I was recruited to one executive position, the chair of family medicine drove me around in her minivan, littered with debris from her kids. It gave us time and topics to talk about, and let us see one another as people and not in a buyer/seller transaction. Our visits to practice sites gave me ideas about what strengths and challenges the organization had. As we drove around, she had trouble finding some of the primary care practice sites. They had poor signage and were in old buildings that were hard to recognize as medical offices. As I commented on that, she told me that the organization had a recent history of undervaluing its owned practices, especially primary care. That gave me some ideas about what was needed, and I was able to use them in subsequent interviews during the day. Turns out the transition to putting primary care front and center in the health system was what they wanted, and I impressed them with my ideas. If the interviews were all conducted in a calm conference room in a hospital building, I would not have had insight into what my job would really be like.

• Just as there needs to be a set of information you want to learn about the candidate, maybe even a formal list of questions, and certain information you want her/him to come away with, the interviewers also need to know the types of questions they can't ask. If you have a human resources department, they should prepare a set of guidelines to this regard, and, if possible, have periodic meetings to review dos and don'ts for interviews. The obvious third rails involve health, marital status, plans for pregnancy, and children. It's generally okay to ask if there is anything that would interfere with their ability to fulfill the role, such as commuting plans.

- There is a technique called "behavioral interviewing" that can be helpful in getting to know and understand a candidate. It involves open-ended questions that encourage the candidate to tell stories about his/her personal experiences. Beyond just helping avoid yes/no answers, it helps uncover skills, experiences, and personal insights. "Tell me about your most difficult management experience in the past year? What did you learn from it? Would you do anything differently?" "What about a challenging patient? Did you reach out to anyone for advice or help?"

I also like to ask about strengths and weaknesses, including why candidates think a particular trait is a strength or a weakness, and how they've worked to improve.

Sometimes a "softball" question turns up an answer that reveals much. I once asked an internal medicine resident interviewing for a primary care position what he thought of the experience he was having in his hospital primary care clinic. "You mean the *primate* care clinic?" he said. After briefly getting an explanation, which basically was "everyone calls it that," I knew there was no reason to continue his visit. Yes, sometimes you politely need to cut the schedule and maybe even explain to the candidate why she/he has struck out.

I've always liked the idea of the lead interviewer, or a trusted recruiter, meeting the candidate at both the beginning and the end of the interview day. That way there can be an introduction to the schedule and to the people who she/he will be meeting. And, at the end of the day, you can set expectations about next steps. If the feedback has been good during the day, you might start a bit of selling and talk about next steps and timeline. I don't like to talk about pay during the interviews, but that should be information (at least the range) the candidate gets during the preliminary phone call. At the end of the day, it may be worthwhile being sure the candidate understands how pay is determined (some don't realize that the range doesn't mean that a newly trained person will be at the top of the range). Earlier, I mentioned that an interview can be the beginning of an employment orientation. This is especially true if you've determined this to be a top person. By talking about how much you value the

Sometimes a "softball" question turns up an answer that reveals much.

traits demonstrated by the candidate and what is needed to be successful in the role, you have a better chance he/she will be making a well-informed decision.

Finally, by all means have a formal, written, interview evaluation completed by all who've met the candidate (including those who give tours or share meals). This has practical value: Offhand remarks, boredom or super-interest, insights about what seemed important to the candidate—all these can help. It's a good idea to be sure the interviewers have the form in advance and that it's filled out quickly after the visit. It can also serve as documentation that explains why someone was hired—or not. In one instance, a senior manager was upset their preferred candidate was not hired. Having the feedback from the interviewers helped explain the decision and took the pressure off me.

There are a lot of parts to an interview and a lot of information to glean. Here's the bottom line for me: I want to know what's in a candidate's heart, what she/he cares about, why she/he is doing what she/he is doing, and what success looks like to her/him. Skills can be seen in a candidate's training, in a CV, and learned from references. There is a saying: "You can teach skills; you can't teach heart." Understanding that can help you decide if the candidate is worth investing in.

REFERENCES

A question that periodically comes up is how valuable is it to check references. It's always done, but does it add anything to the selection process? Asking for and giving a reference has become an issue for many employers due to the potential legal liability of giving information that results in the candidate not getting the job. In fact, some organizations have adopted the position that they'll not provide what had been considered a traditional reference, but will only confirm dates of employment. And it certainly has become the norm for reference information to only be provided in writing. By not having verbal reference information, it's felt that it is less likely for that information to be misused or misconstrued.

What I've seen recently is a process based upon a standardized form—more of a check-the-box approach. You could argue that the whole process has been made so vanilla as to provide little enlightening information.

There will, however, be some instances when checking references can be helpful. If you can find someone to speak with you and help with specific questions (e.g., "She seemed quiet and shy when I met her; what's been the feedback from patients about her communication skills?" Or, "Would you hire her again?" If you hear, "Probably," that might be a red flag.) You might also want to describe the position the candidate is interviewing for and ask if the reference feels that would be a good fit based upon what he/ she has seen of the candidate.

Here's an example of an awkward, maybe over the line, reference check that nonetheless turned up important information. A number of years ago, we were recruiting for an executive suite physician manager and found a candidate working for a nearby, large health services company. He had a good CV and interviewed well. His official references were excellent. However, I was a bit concerned why he wanted our job, which seemed a step down both in responsibility and compensation. I knew one of our former employees with whom I was still friendly worked for that company, possibly in the same unit as our candidate. You probably see where this is going, and I advise you to check with your legal experts about whether you can do what I did. Following this episode, I've always gotten clearance before reaching out to someone not on the official reference list and have gotten conflicting opinions. In this instance, I did call my former colleague and got the inside scoop: The candidate was asked to leave due to performance problems, and was given the good, official reference as part of his settlement, in exchange for a "confidentiality, non-disparagement" agreement. I subsequently told the candidate we would not be hiring him. I didn't explain why, but he knew we had moved on to the reference-checking phase.

Here's a learning: We generally don't spend the time and

energy checking references until we are fairly certain about the candidate, but, if he/she doesn't get the job, he/she now might assume it was because someone he/she thought would provide good comments did not. Should we change the process to ask for references at the same time as we set up interviews? Should we be extra careful not to tip our hand with the candidate before we ask for references? You'll need to think this through with your team, your human resources department, and your legal advisor. This situation became more problematic: I got a call from the executive who had been the supervisor of our candidate. He wanted to know if someone at his company had spoken with me without authorization and told me what I already knew, that there was a confidentiality agreement. Not my finest moment, but I would not confirm that I had an inside source, nor why we decided not to make the hire. It was an ethical dilemma.

The best reference check is the unsolicited comment about a potential clinician hire: "I think she/he is great, I'd hire her/him again, have her/him care for my family (matter of fact, they do care for my family)." That can make you feel confident in your choice. Short of that, a reference will rarely increase the likelihood of her/him being hired, but it may give you valuable pause.

ONBOARDING AND MENTORSHIP

Clearly a great deal of effort goes into recruiting the best candidate for your organization, and you don't want to go through this process more often than necessary. The cost in dollars is significant, as is the time spent. Why, then, don't most employers have a plan to make it most likely that a new hire remains and grows with your organization? There is plenty of advice available for this: books with titles such as *Right from the Start: Taking Charge in a New Leadership Role*[28] and *What Got You Here Won't Get You There.*[29] Still, by some estimates, 20 percent of new hires will be gone from your organization within two years.

One obvious reason is that the fit may not have been right in the first place. The candidate or the organization may not have seen or ignored warning signs. Desperation to fill the spot, or to get a job, may have been the priority. The hope of the candidate that she/he could bend the position to fit his/her needs, or the hiring manager thinking she/he could change the candidate to be what she/he wanted, might not have been a realistic strategy.

Earlier I told the story about the physician who didn't really want to see patients in the hospital and was gone from our group within a few months. Here's some more detail that makes the story even more troubling. During her interview with me, the physician asked if hospital care was a part of the job. She asked why the medical residents at the hospital could not care for our patients. I told her this was not part of our procedure and ethos—we wanted patients sick enough to be in the hospital to be cared for by a physician the patient knew and who knew the patient. Fast forward to the physician's first month in our practice and after one of her first call nights. I received a phone call late one afternoon from a nurse at the hospital asking me why one of our patients hadn't been seen since his admission the evening before. Turns out it was one of my patients, so I went to see him. I dealt with his care and asked him if our physician on-call had been in to see him when he was admitted. I described her, and he said, "No." The next day, I asked the physician if she had gone in while on call. She said, "Yes." When I told her neither the nurse nor the patient had seen her, and there was no chart documentation from her, she admitted she had not. She said she had not realized this was an expectation. I had assumed I'd been clear on expectations and didn't need to review them with her once she was hired. She assumed she could do things her own way and no one would hold her accountable. At that point, I felt I needed to terminate her relationship with our practice—without delay. We paid her for her notice period and told her not to come to work anymore.

Let's assume the person you've hired has a chance to be a good fit. What can you do to optimize his/her chances of success? This moves us to onboarding, including mentorship. I spoke earlier about using the interview process to begin the

Let's assume the person you've hired has a chance to be a good fit. What can you do to optimize their chances of success?

orientation by setting the expectations for the job and by saying what the employer will do to help the new hire fit in. While this didn't work in the case of my earlier story, it often does. At the least, it helps you and the candidate know if the fit will work.

The onboarding and mentoring process starts with setting some expectations. When will the candidate, and potentially the spouse, meet with colleagues and other spouses? Will there be help with finding a place to live, school systems, places to shop, and entertainment? Will there be welcome meetings and/or meals with other staff and with colleagues? What about getting a medical license and other paperwork taken care of—this can be daunting and often takes much longer than expected. More than once we had to push back start dates because licenses and insurance credentialing did not come through—a significant problem if the new hire needs the income, and your team needs the new player.

Our hospital practice assigned a recruiter to the new hires—this person helped them know what was needed when, what to expect, and whom to turn to for help. Since we had a large number of hires each year, we held a two-day, paid, orientation session twice a year. This allowed new hires to meet one another, hear from managers, meet incumbent staff on a social basis, and learn about the basics of the practice, all at once. What is the mission and culture? When will you get paid? Sign up for benefits? Learn about the electronic record? Where are the bathrooms in the hospital? Maybe other clinicians have been hired at the same time for the same practice—this might be the first chance to meet your new partners. Our health system decided to build its own employed hospital physician group. We hired six individuals to begin with and had them be part of the same orientation. They formed a friendship and helped one another get better at their work. As in an earlier example, they were the core of a group that attracted other good clinicians to join them.

Onboarding doesn't stop with the first day of work. There should be follow-up meetings and meals between each new hire and her/his manager. In addition, each new hire should have a mentor. For non-clinicians, this might be an internal or external expert with the time and skills to answer questions and give reassurance. For a clinician, it may be another member of the practice or a member of the clinician management team. It might be that this is done in a confidential fashion, so it's someone the new hire can speak to without fear. Whether such conversations are confidential or not should be made clear to the hire. Often a mentorship is

Onboarding doesn't stop with the first day of work.

voluntary on the part of the employee, and is meant to help that person fit in and grow as a professional. If there is the need for remediation to help the employee meet the expectations of the job, it is not voluntary and is often called "coaching" rather than mentoring. In that case, the coach reports to the employer, and there are often specific goals to achieve.

There is also the informal mentoring process—letting the newbie know that he/she can feel comfortable walking down the hall to ask questions or get reassurance.

In one of my practices, it was the norm for the clinicians to stop by one another's office at the end of the day to see how things had gone. It also was a chance to discuss patients about whom we didn't feel comfortable. We found that all of us had patients for whom we were unsure what to do, and we even had days when we just felt we couldn't make any, let alone the right, decisions. One of the strengths of a group practice is the development of a collective ethos, experiences, and knowledge (more about group practices later in the chapter on Skill #8—Creating the Culture). Our group had almost no clinician turnover, which I attribute at least partly to the support of the initial onboarding and the ongoing peer support.

One day, I had a conversation with a young internist who had trained at the hospital at which we worked. He had been one of the best in his program—in knowledge, work habits, personality, and ethics. He'd gone into solo, private practice, and I asked him how it was going (I secretly hoped he'd want to give it up and join our group). He told me he was scared all the time of doing something wrong with his patients, of making decisions that would hurt them. He was afraid to tell anyone how he felt or ask for help. I described how our group members supported one another by regularly having blame-free, nonjudgmental conversations about patient issues and how to practice better. I encouraged him to speak with the other young clinicians in the community about having regular support sessions. He decided to do that and later became one of the most respected docs in town. Eventually, he organized many of the primary care clinicians into a large group practice without walls, which thirty years later has statewide presence and respect.

BUILDING THE TEAM TAKEAWAYS

- Your team is especially important. You can't do everything yourself, and people won't follow you just because of your title. Take time to think about what kind of team you need and want, and work with others to build it.

- Begin the process with asking the right questions.

- Thoughtful recruiting, interviewing, and reference-checking is key to attracting candidates and assessing the right fit with accuracy.

- Onboarding and mentorship are key to maintaining and continually evaluating fit.

SIX
Skill #3—Communicating

This topic applies to both your own style and also to the expectations of how the team and staff communicate with you and with one another. In the section on dealing with people in Chapter Three, several aspects of communication were covered. Here, the message is that this ability can be learned and improved upon; we shouldn't assume that someone's communication skills on day one are how she/he will always be.

Probably the first step to developing this skill is to communicate! Modeling the behavior for your team and staff is part of it, but so is being explicit about how you'd like to see it done. As a leader or manager, you are now accountable for the behavior of your team—not only what their decisions and actions are, but also how they relate and communicate with others. You don't want to spend a lot of your time and political capital apologizing to others about how you or your team communicate, nor having critical conversations with your team members about something for which you could have better prepared them.

SETTING EXPECTATIONS

Early on in your tenure, it's wise to sit down with your team to go over your expectations about why, when, what, and how to communicate. This is best done conversationally. The best communication is collegial and not top down. You should be explicit about when email is okay, or when texting, phone calls, or face-to-face meetings are preferable, and for what types of issues. Have you been in a situation in which bad news is intentionally left for you as a phone message in your office when the caller knows you aren't there to answer? I have. "I just want to be sure you know I've resigned." Or, "The chief of medicine is mad at me and will probably call you." Is it okay to send an email to someone in an office down the hall, or should you just walk down the hall and leave a note that you'd like to see her/him if her/his office is empty? There should be explicit expectations.

What about evenings, weekends, and other time off? Do you want to be contacted and, if so, for what? Will you be emailing and texting during off-hours? I usually wanted the team to minimize their work during off-hours, feeling the importance of a work-life balance. I stayed away from after-hours emails and told my reports I would only contact them if the issue was important and needed quick attention. This also helped when I was angry about something and my self-imposed limit on emailing gave me time to become more rational first.

One of our medical group managers must have had insomnia, or didn't need sleep, and would email staff at 3 or 4 a.m. I asked him to stop, thinking he should be asleep and not worrying about work at that time. He did stop, but I think what he actually did was write the emails at night and not send them until the next morning. At least he was modeling the behavior we wanted everyone to have.

I can't overemphasize the importance of being explicit with your team and staff about mutual expectations about communication. As touched upon in Part I, a principle I have, and one I expected my reports and colleagues to follow, is "No Surprises." This means I want to hear about things directly from my team, not first from someone elsewhere in the organization or on the outside. This is a corollary to another principle I recommend: If someone is trying to decide whether to tell someone something or not, err on the side of telling it. When your own boss tells you that one of your clinicians is being sued, and she/he hadn't told you first, that's a surprise. When another manager in your health system tells you how great it is that one of your employees is transferring to their department, and the employee hasn't told you, that's a surprise. Most times you are better off sharing information than withholding it (unless it needs to be confidential or is potentially unnecessarily hurtful). By sharing, you are empowering the recipient, letting them know he/she is trusted and you respect his/her feedback to the information. This way you avoid the embarrassing "why didn't you tell me?" when the information (invariably) becomes widely known.

WHAT TO SHARE; WHAT NOT TO SHARE

In every organization I've been a part of, there's been at least one person who was not going to keep information private. Unless you intentionally want something confidential leaked, you might need to be discreet with what you tell that person.

A digression here: Should a staff member tell you that they're looking for another job? More personally, should you tell your boss you are looking for another job? In most instances, I'd say, "Yes." I asked my reports, including clinicians, to tell me if they were on the prowl to change jobs. I let them know that I would be sorry to lose them (though sometimes it was clear the fit was not good and we both were happy they were voluntarily looking elsewhere). Moreover, the amount of time most contracts require for notification of resignation is not adequate for an organization to recruit and onboard a replacement. In the interest of their colleagues (and sometimes their patients), we need more than a few weeks or months to bring a new person on board. When I myself was approached for a position elsewhere, I did tell my boss what I was considering and why. I didn't tell him to leverage my pay or title, but to be respectful of the trust he'd placed in me and so I would not burn bridges. My belief is that there are few secrets, and sooner or later someone will find out—so following the "No Surprises" rubric, it is better to be upfront than to disappoint. The most gracious leaders will be happy or proud that one of their managers has the chance for an even better opportunity.

Here is an example of burning bridges. We had a rheumatologist in our group who'd been with us for a few years. One day I received a request for a reference for a medical license for him in another state (surprise!). I spoke with him, and he claimed he was just applying for it and had no intention to leave (not very convincing). At least at that time we were able to start, quietly, recruiting for a replacement. Six months later, he resigned to go to a job in that other state. A few years later, he contacted us wanting to come back—he didn't realize we didn't trust him enough to hire him again!

Another part of communication skill for a leader/manager is what to say in public, and what to say in private. It's never a good idea to embarrass one of your staff or a colleague in public. When it comes to the folks on my staff I almost always, in public and in private, give them credit for our successes. And I make it a practice to take the responsibility for things that go wrong. It doesn't mean that I don't deal with the staff member about the issue at hand, but I have final accountability in the organization for our failures. (Later on, we'll talk about critical conversations, and we'll give thought to what it means to deal with a bad outcome related to a staff member. For now, I'll say that good people,

CURING PHYSICIAN MANAGEMENT

who try to do the right thing and who can learn from a mistake, are often better at what they do from then on.)

Another aspect of communication is how to relate to other parts of the overall system you're in. I strongly encourage my staff (and try to model) not to attack or bad-mouth others in the organization, either in public or in front of our reports. We don't want to create an us-versus-them mentality at work. Yes, in the short term, having a "common enemy" can help a team bond, but eventually you will need to have common, positive aspirations to sustain you.

I do understand the need to vent at times, so I suggest having a private way for your direct reports to vent to you. Since I would have at least biweekly individual meetings with each of them, that was a good time for that. You'll also get a better idea of what challenges your folks are facing. You might be able to redirect their emotions to positive work, or to explain why something is happening or someone is acting in a certain way, with insights you have as a leader. For example, if we are aware of the financial or staffing stress of another department, we can better understand why they are not open to spending time on issues that are important to us but which are not priorities for them. Everyday professional life is full of examples of internecine rivalries, ambition-driven behavior, and competition for resources. Going on the attack in public, or in front of the wrong people, is almost always wrong, and is best followed by a sincere apology for the behavior, if not also for the sentiment.

It's also worthwhile learning whom you can talk to when you need a confidential ear for advice or to just complain. Is that the person you report to, or is it a coach, a peer, or someone outside the organization?

An example of when communication can go awry: One of my direct reports, a medical director, was accused of being arrogant and condescending to a department chair. This was never said directly to me or to her, but I heard it from several sources. I explained to her that her reputation was somewhat tarnished, and she began to work on not showing that side of herself. But the damage was done. As soon as I was no longer in a position to protect her, she was a goner.

An example of when directly confronting inadequate communication can lead to a good outcome involved the same department chair: I heard from a third party that she had directly contacted one of the clinicians in my group about taking on an academic role in the chair's department. The clinician probably was a good candidate, but was also someone who would be hard to replace in the clinical practice. I immediately and calmly spoke with the chair, explained the problem she was creating, and we agreed on (and henceforth lived by) the idea that we would meet every few weeks and honestly discuss our areas of managerial overlap. This worked well enough that we began to include all our direct reports in similar meetings.

WHERE TO SHARE

We have so many options now of how to communicate—face-to-face, phone, voicemail, text, email, and Zoom. I suggest that face-to-face is the gold standard, but I know it's not always possible. It is particularly important when needing advice or when sharing (good or bad) news. Critical conversations need to happen in person. I've seen important decisions made, or negative feedback given, over email when the sender and receiver of the news are down the hall from one another. Not a good way to be sincere, to provide support, to be honest.

Email can be used to broadly disseminate information. Then it should include an invitation for questions, feedback, and individual or group follow-up. Instead of having multiple email exchanges, there is a point at which a face-to-face or a phone discussion should take place. So many people, including leaders and managers, have fallen into the trap of escalating emotions on email and having something they should not have put into writing accidentally or intentionally widely shared.

> Critical conversations need to happen in person.

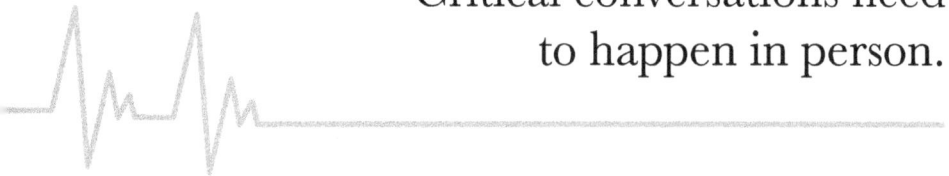

When it comes to communicating with others, whether your team, your peers, or your boss, it is crucial to earn, grow, and preserve your political capital—goodwill. Being trustworthy, and giving trust, bears the fruit of allegiance and cooperation when it is most needed in the future. When your reserves are depleted and your account is emptied, it's hard to rebuild the relationships you need.

COMMUNICATING TAKEAWAYS

- It's easy to make communication mistakes. Work with and listen to others to learn how your communication skills are working.

- Model and set expectations for where, when, and how communications should happen on your team.

- Communication takes many forms: individual, written, electronic, meetings, critical conversations, negotiations. Have an expectation for improvement in communication skills for yourself and for your organization.

SEVEN
Skill #4—Meetings

Ugh, too many meetings![30] When people asked me what I did at work, I often would joke, "I go to meetings so other people don't have to!" This was one of those sardonic, not-without-truth jokes. One of the responsibilities of senior managers is to provide an external face and voice for their work unit, as well as be responsible for the work of their own team (both manage up—representing your team to those outside your work unit— and manage down—being responsible for your own team).

Some business experts estimate there are fifty-five million work meetings in the United States each week, and there are estimates that put the number many times higher. Surveys find that meetings are the least favorite part of work for most people and the biggest perceived waste of time.[31] Seventy percent of senior managers (the people who typically call meetings) don't like going to meetings. Meetings are often repetitious, boring, poorly run, and don't advance your own work.

But the higher up you are in an organization, the harder it is to get anything done without the help of others, and meetings are one of a few ways to align your work with that of other staff. So the issue is how to make meetings more efficient and effective (after you've answered the question of whether, and for whom, the meeting is necessary).

There are several types of meetings: informational, regulatory, agenda-setting, decision-making, review, team-building, showing the flag, and maybe more. They can be phone, video, one-on-one, small or large group, or in-person.

To me, the best meetings I have convened are those at which I didn't need to say much at all. They are the ones for which others were so interested in the topics, had time to think about the issues, and so wanted to contribute to the discussion and outcome, that I just needed to be sure everyone got his/her chance to contribute. How do we make it likely that this will happen?

First let's talk about how to manage a meeting. Sounds really boring, right? Everyone knows how to do this! Then why are there so many bad meetings, after which no one seems to know what was decided and who is doing what next? Why are there so many meetings that participants sit silently through? Or so much hallway complaining after the meeting is over? And with staff often geographically dispersed, how do we know that those on a phone or video meeting are mentally engaged, not multitasking, and have a chance to participate?

Here's a supposedly obvious set of questions about having a meeting:

> The best meetings I have convened are those at which I didn't need to say much at all.

SCHEDULING

Is it a standing meeting that occurs regularly; are you willing to cancel the meeting if there is not much to talk about? What is the expectation of those who will participate? Are call-ins allowable? Does the time/place of the meeting respect the needs of the participants, not just of the presiding manager? How long is the meeting?

Whether in a hospital or medical office, Monday mornings tend to be very busy times. We discouraged having any meetings then. By late Monday afternoon, we were able to hold meetings with my direct reports and with the non-frontline managers to review management priorities for the week. We expected all managers to report on what was going on in their area, what they were working on currently, how that work impacted others at the table, and what they might need help or coordination with. This was not the typical "Morning Report" that medical students, trainees, and academicians may be familiar with, when people are put on the hot seat and expected to perform under stress. It was true information sharing, helping solve problems without blame or public humiliation. During this time, I'd also ask the team what rumors they were hearing, and I would share what I might have heard. If there were significant changes afoot, I wanted folks to hear it from me first and to know how we would be planning for it. Many times perception becomes reality in our minds, causing fear, so if the rumors were unfounded, we wanted to dispel them quickly.

We also held a senior leadership meeting for our team later in the week. This allowed the four or five of us to discuss overarching priorities (e.g., budget, recruiting, negotiations, conflicts with other departments). It helped with bonding and was one venue for venting. It was also where I asked for advice. We created a whiteboard list of major projects and were sure each had a responsible manager and timeline assigned to it, which was updated regularly.

The norm in the world seems to be for meetings to be an hour long. Why is that? Perhaps it's easy to fit into scheduling blocks and to remember, but experience suggests that a meeting will expand into whatever time is allowed for it. You know that your team has other work to do, so you should not be shy about canceling a meeting (preferably in advance) if you know there is nothing new to talk about. At the beginning of a meeting, you might say you'll try to get done early, and follow through if that happens. But, I often noted that the latter suggestion led to attendees unearthing issues they were otherwise hesitant to talk about, and the "shortened" meetings often would run long and be highly productive.

We preferred our meetings to be in-person, at least those not involving clinicians and office/unit staff. That gave everyone the best chance of being engaged and supported.

Who should be invited? Sometimes people don't want to sit through a meeting but they're afraid of being left out or missing something important. One of the chief executive officers I reported to said that most of his management meetings were optional. This was after I told him there seemed to be a lot of meetings with the same core group of people, often covering the same topics, during the course of the week. I then asked why did all the senior leaders show up to every meeting, often seem distracted (more on that soon), and, when they participated, would repeat what they'd said at other meetings? He and I agreed that there was a fear of missing out. And no one wanted to appear to have anything more important to do than attend their boss's meeting.

AGENDAS AND NOTES?

Yes! For general information-sharing meetings, a prepared agenda may not be needed for each meeting; however, if there will be significant discussion topics, then warning folks in advance via email will allow them to give thought (and maybe make extra effort to attend) and be ready to contribute. Notes are also generally a good idea, especially if decisions are made or assignments are given for further work. We've all been to too many meetings during which time was wasted while folks tried to remember what happened in a previous meeting or reargued something everyone forgot was already decided.

I also like to follow up meetings with individual emails to those who had follow-up work to do, especially after meetings with other senior leaders. You're more likely to get your priorities taken care of if they are also priorities for your peers and reports. A good way of cementing those agreements is to put them in writing.

THE TABLE

Have you read about negotiations that have been delayed by arguments over the shape of the table and in which chairs the parties would sit? It is more frequent than one might hope. The talks between North Vietnam and the United States to end the Vietnam War were delayed for months over just that type of disagreement. The North favored a circular table at which all parties, including their partners, the National Liberation Front, would appear to have equal status in the talks. The allies of the United States, the South Vietnamese, insisted on a rectangular table, representing two distinct sides in the conflict. They didn't acknowledge that the National Liberation Front had a separate, legitimate, role in the discussions. The solution, after months, was for the North and South to be at a round table, surrounded by individual square tables for the other parties. Eventually, without much progress through negotiation, the war came to an ignominious end for the US.[32]

My guess is that management issues will not be quite as dire, nor the importance of the table and seating as great, in your management career. But it is still important to consider how they can be set up to optimize the communication and relationships you want to achieve. I'm a fan of having the participants in a meeting be as close to one another as possible, which means a round, oval, or horseshoe table setup. I also suggest putting the person directing the meeting (often the senior leader or manager) in the middle (not at the head). By being in the middle, you're more likely to be heard, can better see body language or when someone is itching to say something, and you're not setting yourself above the others in the meeting (unless it is a time you want to exert your position of power by sitting at the head).

How the meeting and space are structured helps determine who participates and what outcomes you get.

DISTRACTED PARTICIPANTS

Are meeting attendees reading texts and emails on their phones as if something more urgent than the meeting was about to demand their attention? I often sat next to a senior manager who did online shopping on her laptop during the weekly management meeting run by the chief executive officer! To me, it is wise to have explicit guidelines. Cell phones on silent, or turned off, or even surrendered at the door. If on video, establish the expectation that cameras remain on. Asking each meeting participant to report or comment on discussion issues goes a long way to ensuring she/he remain engaged for at least part of the time. If attendees are regularly distracted, it should call into question the value of the meeting.

MEETING TYPES

You should always understand what you want to get from a meeting and knowing the purpose of the meeting is a necessary first step. Here are some meeting types. Remember, a particular meeting may have more than one reason for being, but it is still important to define what those reasons are:

- *Show the Flag*—Usually applies to a senior leader or manager going into the work area, either on foot, or in a meeting room, to stay in touch with what's going on, and probably more so to show that they are interested and care.

- *Informational*—The person running the meeting wants to be sure the participants come away with particular information and messages. This is more often a unidirectional meeting, with time allotted to questions so as to be sure there are no misunderstandings.

If attendees are regularly distracted, it should call into question the value of the meeting.

- *Regulatory*—Meetings that need to occur to check a box and to be sure everyone knows the rules. Examples in health care include meetings mandated by accrediting bodies, such as for corporate compliance. These meetings may be valuable in their own right, but they also require robust attendance, documentation, and reassurance that everyone is paying attention.

- *Agenda Setting*—This type of meeting can overlap with what is often called brainstorming, in which issues are raised, alternatives are considered, and priorities are set. It works better if everyone is engaged and participates.

- *Decision-making*—You'll want to make clear in these what needs to be decided by the end of the time. How many positions to put in the next budget, which candidate to hire, which quality-improvement project to undertake?

- *Review*—The purpose mostly is to hear progress reports on work that is already underway. By scheduling these periodically, it puts pressure on the responsible parties to be working toward the goals being reported upon.

- *Team Building*—All meeting planners should keep this in mind, but some meetings specifically are geared to setting the tone for how the team is important, how people interact with and support one another, and being sure everyone has a chance to see how important she/he is to the group effort.

A special note about phone and video meetings: As organizations have become more widely dispersed, or impacted by the COVID-19 pandemic, and as more work is being done remotely, we need to have a skill set that keeps people engaged and contributing when we are no longer face-to-face. Is everyone paying attention? Is someone annoyed and checked out but we can't see their body language and facial expression? Does someone want to speak and can't find a break in the discourse to cut in? Do some people habitually take up all the air space? I've experienced firsthand what many commentators have written about: the lower barriers to the loss of civility and to personal attacks during remote conversations. The loss of in-person contact, the frustration of not being able to break into a conversation, and the ease of using chat boxes and messages to throw "bombs" requires a new set of rules for what is likely to remain a common type of meeting.

If you are the convener or moderator of a remote meeting, your task is different, and maybe harder, than when everyone is in the same room. There are some positives about video meetings: the use of the Chat or Raise Your Hand functions to know when someone wants to speak or has something to share. Video meetings allow people who have difficulty traveling or who have time limitations to be on an even footing with those on-site. Think about how you want to be treated as a remote meeting participant and what keeps you engaged. I suggest having a set of guidelines, sharing them with your team, and getting their advice and buy-in. Let them know if there will be breaks, if and when there will be time for questions, what the tolerance will be for interruptions, filibustering, and talking over. Continue to have critiques of these meetings, just as you would for those that are in person, to know how to get better.

One final note on meetings: Should you as the leader or senior manager always run the meeting? I'd say not. Sometimes you'll want to intentionally sit to one side and observe; other meetings you might not even want to be in the room. You'll send a message about how much you trust others and how much micromanaging you're into by how you set up your own role. Sometimes there will be a tactical reason for minimizing your role. Years ago, I was part of a small group of managers who knew we had the potential to alienate other managers who we needed to make a decision favorable to us. Instead of leading the meeting and pushing our agenda, we identified one of the quiet, though respected, managers who we knew supported our position but who would normally not speak up. We worked with him to be comfortable taking the lead and supported him before and after the meeting. But during the meeting he did the work. Our goals were achieved, we had new allies, but others believed—and in reality, it was true—that it was their ideas and not ours that won the day.

MEETINGS TAKEAWAYS

- Meetings should be interrogated for their worth and purpose so their functionality is leveraged well and their essential value can be clear to all.

- How meetings are scheduled, how agendas are set, how notes are taken, and even how the tables are arranged are impactful and worthy of your planful attention.

- How to interpret and work with distracted meeting participants.

- Types of meetings and meeting leadership options.

EIGHT
Skill #5—Critical Conversations

You could consider this skill—the ability to have critical conversations—to be another type of meeting, but one that is most often one-to-one, face-to-face, and with a higher degree of urgency and personal impact. Often in this type of meeting, bad news is delivered—news that the manager may feel badly giving and that has a negative impact on the recipient.[33] This skill gets its own chapter because it is an especially important one.

It's most important to be sure your message is clearly conveyed and clearly understood. At the least, you should write down your thoughts so you don't forget what you want to say during a stressful conversation. You may even want to rehearse your initial comments. I've seen conversations after which the principals don't agree on what the outcome was ("I didn't think I was fired"; "I didn't think I was being blamed").

Please maintain some flexibility in your thinking because, not infrequently, the plan going into the meeting changes during the conversation. This is not necessarily bad—it may be that new facts come to light—"Yes, I've been late recently, but my spouse is away to care for a relative and I need to get the kids on the school bus." Or you realize that the employee has a good heart, is sincere, and commits to an actionable improvement plan. There is a concept currently much in favor in health care and elsewhere to support a "just culture." It's an effort to differentiate human error from at-risk behavior and from reckless behavior. For the first, the path is to console; for the second, to coach; and for the last, to discipline. There's evidence that someone can become a more valued employee through coaching. So, it may be worth the effort, at least for the first occasion, to gear the critical conversation toward improvement and not toward reprimand or termination.

On the other hand, though, there may be a time when you conclude that the effort and angst that you and the employee will need to go through means it just won't work out. When that's your conclusion, after careful consultation with other managers (including your human resources advisors), it is often best to move toward a separation.

A few words about the importance of partnering with the human resources team or advisors: When you are making a decision that will significantly impact a staff member, you'll need to be sure of your organization's policies and procedures, legal requirements and processes, as well as the operational and ethical considerations. As much as possible, I would not only ask the HR staff for guidance, but would

It's most important to be sure your message is clearly conveyed and clearly understood.

partner with them in delivering the message to the employee. It often is valuable to have a collaborating witness should the conversation become heated. And it is sometimes better to tag team with someone who can help during the stressful moments and also answer questions about process (including potential appeal or alternative positions, compensation, and benefits). Having said this, it is important for you, as the senior manager and leader, to take the lead and the responsibility for the decision. It is never good to act as though it wasn't your idea or blame others for the ultimate decision. With this type of decision, as well as others, once you act as though you don't have responsibility and power, others will begin to believe that is indeed the case and you will lose credibility and respect.

CRITICAL CONVERSATIONS TAKEAWAYS

- You need to be able to have hard, critical conversations.

- Flexible thinking will allow you to be open to critical conversations having different outcomes than you originally envisioned.

- Remember to include HR in certain circumstances.

NINE
Skill #6—Negotiation

One would think that decades after the publication of *The Art of Negotiating*,[34] by Gerald Nierenberg, and *Getting to Yes*,[35] by Roger Fisher and William Ury, that the ability to negotiate in good faith, by honest brokers, as a way to increase value would be universally embraced. Yet very often we hear people speak of "zero-sum negotiation" or "games," in which the gain by one party means a loss by another. We see the terminology of war or sports, in which there are winners and losers, applied to deeply personal relationships, such as clinician and patient, peer and peer, manager and staff. Many who have studied negotiating see that viewing the "pie" as something that can be enlarged for all to share is the preferable outcome.

Adam Grant from the Wharton School of the University of Pennsylvania identifies negotiators as "takers"—those who try to optimize their own gains despite the consequences for the other party, and "givers"—those who try to optimize the outcome for all concerned. He goes further: "But now there's a science of the deal, with decades of evidence on what separates great negotiators from their peers... Being a giver may actually be a sign of intelligence." He continues: "The smarter people were, the better their counterparts did in the negotiation. They used their brainpower to expand the pie, finding ways to help the other side that cost them nothing…. The most successful negotiators cared as much about the other party's success as their own…. They didn't declare victory until they could help everyone win."[36] As we spoke about the nonviolence of Gandhi being a proactive force for change, likewise the desire to benefit all in a negotiation is not a sign of meekness or lack of intellectual integrity.

It isn't hard to understand that the desire to win could be part of the persona of a health care leadership that has traditionally been dominated by well-educated, striving men. Going back to our discussion of how medical education can shape and/or reinforce certain ways of behaving, those take-charge, "I know what I'm doing" traits can be reassuring and even lifesaving in certain situations. But they can be off-putting and destructive when wielded by managers and leaders.

One of the physician executives I worked for early in my career took pride in his ability to negotiate with other physicians and their practices. He was not new to negotiating, and he knew he needed to have a firm grasp of the data. The people he was negotiating with often did not have the same level of experience, nor the same access to data, and they sometimes were misled by his flattery of their clinical ability and by their own egos (remember the flaw of physicians thinking knowing how to be a doctor means they know how to do everything?). Our executive came back boasting about the one-sided deals he was able to win. But all deals have an end point. When he left, and I and others needed to maintain relationships and negotiate new contracts, we were hit by the backlash. The people who had "lost" in the previous negotiation realized they'd been taken advantage of and demanded better deals.

Taking advantage of who you're negotiating with is not a good way of forming a long-term relationship, one in which each party has a stake in making the deal work. The goal should not be to be on different sides, but for everyone to be on the same side. Does this sound Pollyannaish? Sure does. Can you always make everyone happy? No. Is it worth trying? Yes!

A few broadly applicable principles of negotiation are as follows:

- Know what your options are and how much authority you personally have before you enter into the negotiation. Understand how important a successful outcome is to your organization. Talk to all your internal stakeholders to get their ideas and priorities.

- When you begin working with your counterparts, be upfront about why a negotiated deal is important to you and be sure they tell you what success will look like to them.

- Decide who is to participate in the negotiation, who the decision-makers are, who are advisors, who are kept informed, and who won't be involved.

- Share all the data: Holding back important information does not build trust. Always assume that there will be no secrets. Someone will find out "secrets" in some way, even if all parties have signed confidentiality agreements.

- Set a schedule for discussions, stick to it, and have a timeline for making decisions.

- Prioritize broad goals before details and decide if you're willing to give up on the latter to achieve the former.

- Know when the deal is good enough and when to walk away.

- Understand the alternatives, what's called in management jargon, the BATNA—the best alternative to a negotiated agreement. If you can't make a deal that works for both parties, what alternatives does each have? Be planning throughout for what you'll do next if there is not a deal.

- Strive to create a trusting, respectful relationship, one that can be built upon. Bad contracts can be remedied or will eventually expire. Bad relationships will cause constant pain, are hard to fix, and may not endure (or you may be stuck with them but wish they went away).

- Above all, have some common sense. Using data and learning new skills doesn't get you far if you can't read and adjust to the situation, pay attention to the emotions across the table, and be willing to adjust your positions on the fly.

CLINICIAN-PATIENT NEGOTIATIONS

Let's talk about different negotiating situations, beginning with the clinician-patient relationship. You might not think there is much negotiation in this. The clinician tells the patient what they should do, and the patient follows instructions, right? When I was a young physician that was what I assumed would happen. When something didn't turn out "right," it wasn't my fault. The patient wasn't listening, wasn't smart enough, or was noncompliant. Lack of discussion, of understanding what each party was trying to achieve, of agreeing together on goals and steps to those goals, of explaining and offering choices were generally not considered to be part of the clinician-patient relationship.

In recent years, a wealth of research has demonstrated the shortcomings of those attitudes and approaches. The idea of shared decision-making has been studied and verified as valuable in creating relationships and being effective at motivating and changing behavior.[37] It is important to understand what the patient values, what they fear, what they want to make better. As studies have shown, when a clinician stops a patient from talking in a mean time under twenty seconds, thinks she/he has heard enough, and knows enough to tell the patient what to do, it can lead to a poor outcome. Hence the general failure to achieve behavior changes about smoking, diet, exercise, medication compliance, preventive testing, etc. Now young clinicians are versed in (and hopefully are following) the precepts of active listening, partnering, and behavioral motivation. Is this starting to sound like a negotiation? The clinician and patient sharing what they know, and the patient being able to say what they value, leads to a plan that potentially works better and pleases both.

A fairly simple example of a clinician-patient negotiation is the approach to prescribing antibiotics in nonurgent situations. Hopefully, most reading this are aware that the world has a problem with the spread of drug-resistant bacteria, at least in part due to the overprescribing of antibiotics for viral or other self-limiting conditions (the United States Center for Disease Control estimates that one-third of antibiotic prescriptions are unnecessary).[38] Clinicians often admit that such use is unscientific and detrimental. But they rationalize that it's what the patient wants; if a prescription isn't written, then the patient will go elsewhere and get one. But studies don't bear this out. In fact, having a discussion, providing explanations, and offering alternatives often result in fewer inappropriate prescriptions. Here's what we tried in our primary care practice: "I don't see something here that an antibiotic will help, since they treat bacterial infections and not viruses. But things can change, and I don't want you to be caught with a worsened problem needing to seek care again. Here's a prescription for an antibiotic for common respiratory bacteria. If over the next few days, you develop a higher fever, or your mucus darkens, fill it and let me know afterward what you've done. Until then, here are the self-care things you can do to feel better and allow your body to heal itself." Our own follow-up and medical studies have shown that only about a quarter of the patients will fill the prescription.[39] A win-win: I've helped the patient and helped decrease the spread of resistant organisms. The patient now has knowledge and autonomy. Did they come for a drug, or was it for reassurance and to just feel better?

NEGOTIATING COMPENSATION

Another type of negotiation for a clinician manager/leader is agreeing on compensation with a new hire or an incumbent employee. There are many things that can go wrong in this process, and it's easy for misunderstandings to grow into antagonism. I'm not going to go into detail on all the background issues. If you work as part of a larger organization, you'll have the benefit of someone dedicated to helping you with compensation, and you likely won't have a lot of flexibility with any particular employee. How important is the hire or staff member for your organization; how scarce is the skill set you're trying to fill; are you recruiting nationally against higher income localities; what's the current pay scale; will you be disadvantaging other staff members by paying a new person more than an incumbent; are you respecting diversity and equity values?

What I'm going to suggest are not hard-and-fast rules, proven by study. They're just ones that I'm comfortable with and seem to take some of the stress and disappointment out of the process, at least for me.

I am a fan of being upfront and honest with someone applying for a position. I don't want to waste his/her and my time only to find out we can't agree on financial terms. I know some will try to win the heart of the candidate and hope he/she will then "accept" an offer. And I've had some candidates tell me a pay range was acceptable to them only to try later to get more (after they think they've won my heart?).

I don't want someone to take a position, or to remain in one, when he/she has a better opportunity, just because I've outbid another employer. All too often in our fragmented, contentious, dispassionate health care business world, people validate their own worth by what they are paid. I would almost always rather have people on the team who value their work and colleagues and doesn't put dollars at the top of their list.

I've also found that once someone is unhappy with his/her compensation, it's very hard for him/her to get over that. Often, it's just the tip of the unhappiness iceberg. Convincing someone to join your team, or to remain, based upon money, is a fraught victory.

So I will tell candidates what the pay range is, how we decide where to place a new hire on that range, and how to expect advancement (and, no, this is not Lake Wobegon and everyone is not "above average"). For incumbents it's much the same—not what others make, but what the range is and how the work expectations and performance fit in.

I will be more flexible with non-salary issues (not "benefits," which must be standardized, whether they are pension, insurance, or time off). But start date, tuition reimbursement, and work schedule (as long as it fits into the needs of the team) are negotiable. And I will advocate for higher compensation when the market or performance warrants. I will do this not just for the individual but for all those affected. If we need to pay primary care candidates more because the market is moving faster than our benchmarks, then we should be paying our incumbents accordingly. Remember, there will be no secrets—your incumbents will likely find out what the newbies are being paid. You can't be disingenuous and then expect to be trusted.

In my management life there was often a larger, more risky type of negotiation, which involved the hiring of a group of physicians. Most often this is a negotiation between a health care system and a private medical group (though it can also be a merger of groups or a contractual relationship between a group and an insurance company). The likelihood is that if you are a physician in management, or a manager of physicians and practices, this is something you'll find yourself undertaking at some point.

Here's a real-life example of a high-stakes negotiation that was successful, after much pain and compromise, and had a big reward for all parties. It created a foundation for the future of the physicians, their group practice, the health system, and the community.

Our community had a tradition of specialty physicians being in private practice and being part of large groups with almost no competitive practices in their field. One particular group of about fifteen physicians was having trouble managing itself. There were several internal factions. The older docs, the founding partners of the practice, were generalists in their field. The younger docs, who were coming up for partnership, had different lifestyle and financial expectations, and most often were sub-subspecialists. Another split, mostly along age-fracture lines, was that the younger physicians did most of the hospital care, including caring for patients in the intensive care units. As for many groups, this one had invested heavily in their office real estate. This was part of the retirement plan for the older physicians, and they expected the younger ones to buy into the real estate and buy the senior physicians out, when it came time for their retirement. However, with the onset of the great recession in 2008, the real estate sank in value, and the younger physicians didn't want to invest in a depreciating asset. The younger physicians spent much of their time in the hospital versus the office and didn't see an office as a necessity. They saw the potential of much of their income coming from the health system and they felt the higher insurance reimbursements they received for acute care were subsidizing the incomes of the older physicians.

This group was in danger of imploding, with some of the older clinicians thinking of early retirement, and some of the younger ones starting to interview for positions in other communities. The health system was worried; remember, there were no other practices able to fill the needs it was filling. It would take a long time for the system to create a new practice of employed physicians if they lost this group. There was no guarantee this could be done with the same level of quality that the current group was providing the community.

The group leadership, representing the two factions, came to the health system for help. I was assigned to lead the team to work with them. Here are the steps we took:

- I worked with my medical group management team to create a value proposition, outlining why it was important for patient care, and how it would work financially, if we employed the physicians. Having done this before, we already had codified a way of looking at this. We also had already set up a process for the mechanics of negotiating, hiring, acquiring, onboarding, and managing a practice.

- I went to the health care system's chief executive officer and the chief financial officer to be sure I had their support in principle for employing the physicians, and, if need be, to acquire their practice assets, including their office real estate.

- I then went to the senior management team to let them know the risks and benefits and the value proposition and outlined the process. I made sure they were comfortable with the goals and process. If someone was not, we spent time working out our differences. This was especially true for the health system medical director for specialty care and for the chief financial officer. We established a standard of confidentiality (it is not a good idea to have this process a subject of gossip and public misunderstanding) and of regular check-ins.

- We created a team to be "at the table." It included—in addition to the medical group operations manager and me—senior representatives from human resources, compensation, legal, and finance. We intentionally did not include on the team the medical director for specialty care (with the permission of the CEO and the chief medical officer). We felt that person was too close to the individual physicians in the group, and was more likely to say, "Give them what they want," than to look for ways to meet the needs of all parties. We committed to regular communication with that person, including input in designing our positions, discussions before and after negotiating sessions, and being an equal partner in the future management and planning for the practice.

- Only then did we have the first working session with the group leaders. We did that after explaining to them what we expected at that meeting: an introduction of both teams; a review of the current status of the practice, including the internal dynamics; a detailed discussion of what both parties wanted out of the negotiations; a frank conversation about how hard this would be; and what the time commitment, timeline, and scope of issues to resolve would be. I told them there would be angry moments and meetings. Anger and disagreement would extend to the clinicians and health system managers, who were not part of the negotiation, but our goal was important enough that we would accept that anger and not let it prevent a successful negotiation.

- Sometimes during these types of negotiations, additional expertise needs to be consulted, or brought into the room. Sometimes a physician practice wants its attorney to be part of their team. That is acceptable, and, if so, if one attorney would not be available for a session, we would exclude the other attorney. For this particular negotiation, the practice elected not to have its attorney present to save themselves fees but shared all meeting minutes and documents with her.

- Other types of outside experts might be consultants in fair market value compensation, real estate brokers (to determine the value of the office space), and asset evaluators (for equipment).

- Each meeting had an agenda and goals for what progress we wanted to make.

- We kept notes of all meetings, leaving out mentions of anger, posturing, etc., and distributed the notes to each party to be sure we knew what we had covered, agreed upon, and what outside work we needed to do. To keep things moving, it is important that work is done between sessions. All too often we fall into the trap of only doing work on a matter while in a meeting. It's also important to have notes for each team to use so they can accurately report back to their constituents. Moreover, this way if anyone misses a meeting, she/he knows what is happening without causing delays at the next session.

- Yes, there was anger. Sometimes someone didn't get what she/he wanted from the health system, or the health system representatives thought the practice to be unreasonable in its requests. Sometimes the two factions of the practice were at odds over who was getting more of what it wanted.

This negotiation went on for four months, with mostly weekly team meetings, but sometimes with individual conversations to clarify or iron out issues. At that point, we had most of the general terms agreed upon and could be sure the health system and practice partners were ready to sign off on the framework of the final deal. We were able to set a target date (two months off) that allowed each individual clinician and his/her staff (since we were able to offer health system employment to most) to review the compensation and benefit package and meet with the health system human resources team. We provided the attorneys with the terms so they could draw up documents and move forward on leases and asset acquisition.

Were all the practice clinicians and staff happy? No. Neither were all the health system folks, especially in finance. The latter couldn't get over the fact we would now be paying salary and providing benefits to people to work in our hospital, whereas previously those folks were directly compensated by insurance reimbursements provided without financial risk to the system.

As the day neared for the clinicians to sign their agreements, some tried to use what they hoped was personal leverage to get a better deal for themselves. One person was persistent enough to threaten not to sign on unless we gave him a higher salary. He wasn't a great player in the practice previously, so the practice leaders weren't ready to fight for him. After explaining that we were not going to change his compensation as it seemed to fit with the model we were using for the entire practice, I let him resign. A few weeks later, the practice manager told me the physician had reconsidered and would accept our offer. We signed him on. A lesson here—he was unhappy from the start, as he'd been prior to our acquisition, and became disruptive in the office. Eventually, I needed to tell him it was time to go. If someone is unhappy over money, it's hard to convert him/her to being part of the team. I probably should not have given myself permission to sign him on after his initial tirade.

Years later, the practice continues to thrive. Some of the older clinicians took advantage of the security offered by employment to plan their orderly retirement. The strength of the health care system made recruitment of new talent possible, especially of younger physicians who, in general, are not that interested in private practice. The ability to provide dedicated and skilled staff for the critical care and acute units was improved: We were able to have full-time access to

We used the negotiation as a model for how a successful, long-term partnership could, and did, work.

critical care specialists, something the private practice was not willing to provide. Most of the clinicians and the practice manager have remained with the health system, some taking on leadership roles.

It would be great—and not possible—to say that all our negotiations worked out so well. They have been a tremendous investment of time and money. But those that came to fruition, which most did, did so because of a structured approach—one that recognized the value of the practice and the individuals, that respected their needs, helped them to save face and maintain at least some control over their professional lives. And we used the negotiation as a model for how a successful, long-term partnership could, and did, work.

NEGOTIATION TAKEAWAYS

- Take some time to learn best practices and skills.

- Be thoughtful about your team; don't do this alone (unless it is a patient-clinician "negotiation"). Even if it's dealing with the compensation of staff or clinicians, be sure you are clear on your options.

- Do pre-work to get everyone on board with the plan.

• Look for ways to create value for each party.

• Know what your alternatives are and "when to hold them and when to fold them"— that is, when to walk away from the table.

• Don't be afraid of emotions, but always come back to your mutual goals. Try to attack problems and issues, not people.

TEN
Skill #7—Decision-Making

You've probably realized by now that there is significant overlap, or complementarity, between many of these skills. That also goes for this one—decision-making—which could easily have been included under "Skill #2—Building the Team," "Skill #5—Critical Conversations," and "Skill #6 – Negotiation."

A sentiment attributed to John F. Kennedy is that there are two kinds of decisions a president can make—a bad one and a worse one. Maybe this idea is a bit sarcastic, but there is something we can learn from it about decisions.

Some decisions don't have good outcomes for anyone involved. There are also some decisions that can have a favorable outcome even if they were based upon faulty reasoning. If a patient is given an antibiotic for a cold and gets better, it probably wasn't the "right" decision, but it can appear as though it was, at least to the patient. Anecdote is a powerful force for both patients and clinicians and can override what may be a more scientific approach.

When an outcome is good despite what may appear as a faulty process to an objective observer, it reinforces the further use of that bad process (e.g., we might hire someone who turns out to be great despite not having gone through a thorough vetting process). Earlier, I shared the saying, "Even a blind squirrel can find nuts." Though I never researched to see if that is true, we can still appreciate the sentiment.

BEING PREPARED TO MAKE A DECISION

Decision-making involves many of the same steps as hiring a new team member: understanding what the goals are, the short- and longer-term needs; what information is needed to arrive at a favorable conclusion; thinking through the benefits of an option, as well as understanding the risks.

By spending time on the downsides of an option, it does not necessarily mean you or someone else is taking a negative position. It is important to know what to expect so you can be prepared to take steps to make it more likely the decision will work out. An example of this might be the selection of a new team member. Maybe you've identified some weaknesses in that person, but you see plenty of potential. Instead of deciding not to make the hire, you might go forward, but set up mentoring and monitoring, as well as adjusting the initial work expectations to help the person get established.

An important part of decision-making is to define who will make a particular decision. It is in the interest of the senior leader to minimize the number of decisions to make herself or himself. This may seem paradoxical, but it follows the logic that the higher up in an organization a person might be, the

An important part of decision-making is to define who will make a particular decision.

harder it is for that person to get things done by herself or himself, and the more important it is to empower others to have responsibility and accountability. Once the goals and culture of your team or organization are established, the clinician leader needs to set an expectation about which types of decisions he/she just needs to be informed about, when he/she wants to give advice, and when he/she needs to be actively involved. It also means backing up the decisions made by your team and not casting blame should things go wrong.

Here's an example of just such a misstep in setting expectations. Our clinician management team was working on a compensation model for one of our specialty groups. We had discussed transitioning away from volume-based to quality-based pay; I thought that would be what the model would reflect. The team thought they had final decision-making authority. What the team presented to me was almost entirely a productivity model—way off my target. I needed to override its plan (fortunately done in a private meeting), but doing so was embarrassing to the manager, who'd put in most of the work on it. We ended up having a strained relationship for some time afterward.

We should remind ourselves that decision-making in management is not always the same as in clinical medicine. A similarity, though, is that there is the need for pragmatism. You might need to make a decision with incomplete information. For example, in clinical medicine, you might choose an antibiotic for bacterial pneumonia without the results of a sputum sample (though guided by data-driven guidelines). In management, you might not have the data to know what the consumer wants. This should not paralyze you. A primary care practice I was managing was working a 9 a.m. to 5 p.m. schedule Monday through Friday. We served a working population, including many young families. As the manager I convened a group of clinicians to discuss extending our office hours to include early, late, and weekend times. Some clinicians objected, saying we didn't have the data to know that was something the consumers wanted. But we went ahead anyway. I thought it was not worth the effort and time to pre-study, but we could get feedback once we were rolling along and adjust as needed. The new appointment availability was a big satisfier for our patients. The data that supported it was evident in the demand for appointments. We did modify the

Decision-making in management
is not always the same as in
clinical medicine.

plan by decreasing Sunday hours, but ended up beefing up the staffing on Saturdays. Change can be scary and disruptive, and sometimes people will hide behind a demand for data to slow down a decision process. In this case, as sometimes happens, you'll need to push ahead anyway—especially if the decision supports the values and goals you've established (in this case, exceptional access to care).

DECISION FATIGUE

Decision paralysis or fatigue is a real thing, and there have been many studies looking at the causes and how to deal with it. It can come from pressures from the external environment (trying to please many different people and constituencies) or can be part of your personality profile.[40] It can come from having too little data or too much. It can be a result of not having good options or of having too many. On the latter point, it's been shown that trying to sort out from a large number of options (in regular life, an extensive restaurant menu, for example) can result in what's now called a "fear of missing out"—FOMO. The consequences in the restaurant are probably not very great; if you end up with a bad meal, you could make a different choice next time. But if you've hired the wrong person, the downside can be much more troublesome.

For most management decisions, you can take the time to get advice from others and measure what you want to achieve against your goals and needs. It is also important to realize you may not be able to heed all the advice you're given—sometimes it will be conflicting. And you need to set a time limit on when a decision needs to be made. "By the end of the month, we will hire Dr. X if there are no better candidates." Or, "If there are no better candidates by the end of the month, I will let Dr. X know we are not hiring her and will reopen the recruit."

The straw-man approach can be used when it becomes too hard for individuals or groups to come to grips with making decisions. The team may not have as much information as you do or enough time to prioritize the decision process. Maybe team members are used to a cultural paradigm—say, the importance of consensus—which cannot always be achieved. Or they don't like to "hurt the feelings of," or disagree with, their colleagues or friends. When it doesn't seem that others can get off the starting line, or they are too paralyzed to move along, a straw man outlining a path, or a few alternative paths, can get them started. Remember to tell the team that it can throw darts at the proposal and change it—it's okay if it's a stupid idea, or the stupidest idea; we just want to get folks thinking and reacting. Who knows! Very likely the team will come up with something better.

DECISION-MAKING TAKEAWAYS

- Decisions can, and usually should, be planned for.

- Decision fatigue is real; work through it by setting time limits for decisions, getting advice but knowing when to stop asking for input; and exploring "straw man" options.

ELEVEN
Skill #8—Creating the Culture

"If you can't maintain your culture during the down times,
then you don't really have a culture."

—STEVE KERR, *championship-winning coach of the Golden State Warriors*

You may have heard the expression, "Culture eats strategy for lunch, every day." Not particularly scientific, but it gets right to the point—what people feel and believe, what's important to them, and what they're comfortable with can easily overwhelm rational thought and planning. Culture can be a driver of success, as Coach Kerr relates, or it can get in the way of success.

Culture is more formally defined as how a group of people think, their attitudes, and beliefs. It's how they behave when no one is watching or telling them what to do.

ASSESSING THE CULTURE

As a new manager or leader, or even as someone who is experienced but new to a role or organization, it is well worth your time to observe and learn about the culture of which you're now a part. For the confident and enthusiastic leader who comes with a set of changes (more on the change process in the next section) and plans, to not know how folks behave and interact will be at least frustrating, if not highly problematic, as she/he tries to implement a plan.

Culture may have developed because of prior management decisions, the origin of which and reason for which are long forgotten. Culture may have been created by an individual or group whose behavior as positive or negative role models taught others how to prosper, or just to survive, in the work environment. It may have come from other places people had worked or trained, even from their families, and superseded or overwhelmed whatever the previous culture had been. Or the culture may have arisen purely in a laissez-faire manner, by people who didn't give much thought to the concept, but just behaved and worked the way they thought they should.

There may be nothing wrong with the culture, or that might be your opinion, unless and until it comes time to change something or when things are going poorly. A concept in change management is the force-field analysis: What are the reasons and momentum to make a change versus what are the reasons and inertia to leave things alone? At the top of the list of resistance to change is culture, and at the top of the list of things that may need changing is culture.

CHANGING THE CULTURE

Culture cannot be changed by memo or fiat. Understanding the current culture is needed, not to tell people what the new one is, but to know where the starting point is for your work. The path to a new culture includes having a vision, communicating it, demonstrating and reinforcing and persisting in new behaviors, and, if possible, showing evidence that the new state is an improvement over the old.

Do not start out by saying the culture needs to, or will, change. But do create the systems, policies, and procedures that will result in new behaviors. Those behaviors, over time, with reinforcement and persistence, will become the new norm, and eventually the new culture. It may take some time, even a year or two, but you'll know that it has happened when you don't have to tell people what to do anymore; they just do it. And when new team members join, they are quickly swept into the cultural flow. This is not the same as "group speak," meaning everyone thinks the same or feels/believes the same (unless that is the culture you want, which I don't recommend). The type of culture I prefer is questioning, creative, participatory, individually self-fulfilling by contributing to the overall success, and aspiring to achieve the goals of the team and organization.

Do not start out by saying the culture needs to, or will, change. But do create the systems, policies, and procedures that will result in new behaviors.

To summarize, here are key points in developing a culture that contributes to success:

- Know what the current culture is (maybe it's fine already and you just need to respect it and not try to bend it to your will).

- Have a vision for the desired future state.

- Plan for the system and processes that will need to be in place to achieve the vision. Strive for vigorous input and buy-in to the vision, system, and processes (not passive acceptance).

- Develop a timeline for the steps to be taken.

- Be patient. Let each step have time to work (or to find out what needs to be modified).

- Be ready to intervene if there are naysayers out to protect their own interests or power. Be ready to step aside for other opinion leaders and role models to take the reins (in fact, work actively to identify and empower those folks).

While you are visioning the culture changes you wish to make, here are some examples of problematic cultures and norms of behavior:

• Team members or other managers who are afraid to speak up because different opinions and honest disagreements are not valued.

• Priority is given to the wants of staff rather than to the needs and preferences of the customers. A few real-life examples: Telling patients that if they're late by X minutes they need to reschedule, without regard to the reason for their care, the reason for their lateness, or for how inefficiently and late the practice itself operates. Or allowing each clinician the ability to dismiss a patient from her/his practice for his/her own reasons and also prevent that patient from receiving care from anyone else in the practice (lest it cause embarrassment for the first clinician).

• Adhering to the unspoken (and culture is most often unspoken) pecking order that physicians (white coats) should be more powerful than other managers (suits) and deferred to when there are differences of opinion.

• Believing that medical care, and especially how medicine is practiced, has reached a utopian state, and improvement is not worth the time nor effort. It has often amazed me that clinicians have accepted that there are new and better ways of treating many diseases, but not that we could learn, adopt, and adjust to new ways of delivering care.

When those types of cultural dynamics can be avoided and changed, here are some examples of more successful types of cultures that can arise:

- A medical group that made several key physician hires, who became thought leaders and role models and attracted many more like-minded clinicians and multiple support staff members, without (maybe, despite) the work of management.

- A medical practice in which each clinician felt she/he was an independent practitioner and controlled her/his own staff members, that suffered from high staff turnover and low patient satisfaction, went on to become a team of mutually supportive members, focusing on patient outcomes and satisfaction, with a staff that made the extra effort to help one another.

- A management team that would argue an issue for an hour, could come out of the room respecting one another with a shared understanding and commitment to the path forward.

GROUP CULTURES—PROS AND CONS

One of my foundational management tenets is that groups and teams underlie organizational success. Leadership and management help create the culture of the team and then need to minimize the control they exert. In health care, the success encompasses the patients/consumers/and population served and the satisfaction and commitment of the team members.

Some cultures and organizations operate on an "every person for themselves" principle—like a baseball team of individual "stars" each doing their own thing. What I've been advocating for is the type of team or group that expects individuals to work together toward common goals.[41] But I want to be explicit in laying out what in everyday practice "team" means, and why it might not be for everyone.

A well-functioning group culture:

- Provides for the sharing of expertise, knowledge, and responsibility;

- Provides a framework for taking risks and for innovating;

- Raises the standards of performance—seeing examples of how people do things differently and sometimes better, supporting a quest for the "greatest common denominator";

- Gives the collective more influence than that of any individual;

- Aligns goals and efforts, making it more likely things can get done;

- Shares the work burden;

- Allows individuals to share in the success of others and of the group as a whole.

Here are some things that can be viewed as downsides to a team culture, even if the group is well functioning:

- A sacrifice of the ability to take individual actions;

- Words and actions are subject to scrutiny and potential criticism;

- More spoken and written rules (except when culture takes over) that regulate norms of behavior and engagement;

- Shared influence and power;

- Homogenization, including moving to the "least common denominator" of performance;

- Group thought, diminishing the role of creativity;

- Lowered personal status.

For some individuals, the downsides outweigh the positives; for them, your team may not be the right place.

Once again, the way to optimize the positives is to have shared goals, to be planful, to communicate, to respect, and to be willing to share your status, influence, and indeed, leadership, with a high-functioning culture and team.

The way to optimize the positives is to be have shared goals, to be planful, to communicate, to respect, and to be willing to share your status, influence, and indeed, leadership, with a high-functioning culture and team.

CREATING THE CULTURE TAKEAWAYS

- Don't even begin to think about changing the culture before thoughtfully assessing what the current culture is and understanding how it got that way, as best as you can.

- What well-functioning group cultures can look like, as well as cultures to be wary of.

- Your life will be easier if the culture of the organization supports well-intentioned, knowledgeable, independent team members and behavior. All your actions should contribute to that culture.

TWELVE

Skill #9—Change Management

"It is not the strongest of the species that survive, nor the most intelligent, but the most responsive to change."

—CHARLES DARWIN

"Better is good."

—PRESIDENT BARACK OBAMA

You've heard the expression—"if it ain't broke, don't fix it." Well, my advice is to remove that thought from your mind. To think that everything is perfect, that nothing better can be done, to ignore that progress often comes in small building steps is hubris, and hubris should not be part of the personality of a leader. Yes, the time to change or fix something may not be now, maybe it's not the current priority, but that doesn't mean processes and systems, and yes, people, can't be better. Douglas Adams, the creator of *The Hitchhiker's Guide to the Galaxy* and of the succeeding books, once said (I paraphrase), "Why do we think human beings are at their highest level of evolution?" The same can be said for health care systems and medical practices!

Change—planful, managed change—is the tool that allows us to not only "fix" things, but to make them better. It can be painful. Change in organizations often fails. Some say that 70 percent of change efforts are abandoned within the first year. So it is worthy of serious thought before beginning the work of change. Let us take time here to discuss it.

GRIEVING CHANGE

Many of you will be familiar with the five stages of grief model developed by Dr. Elisabeth Kübler-Ross. I see many aspects of the change process closely paralleling grieving. This is not to trivialize the emotional impact of tragedy, upheaval, and death, but to help us understand how significant change may be experienced by those it impacts. Kübler-Ross named the five stages as:

Denial—evidenced by avoidance, confusion, shock, fear, panic.

Anger—At ourselves, the person or thing we've lost, any possibly responsible people or entities, with frustration, irritation, and anxiety.

Depression—Feeling hopeless and helpless, overwhelmed.

Bargaining—Looking for meaning, looking for help.

Acceptance—Exploring new relationships and behaviors, planning, coping, accepting, and moving forward.

People move at different rates, and sometimes in different sequences, through the steps. Sometimes a step seems to be skipped. Sometimes someone will become stuck in one state and can't move on.

But just as there are ways to help with grief, there are ways to work with change. Kübler-Ross's model tells us that help flows from information and communication, through emotional support, to guidance and direction. Just as the lived stages of grief may not follow the textbook model, neither may the ways of dealing with it. Like with grief, the process of change for individuals is influenced by past experiences and by the support provided by their friends and families. Organizations can also go through grief. For an organization, grief is the sum total of trauma or setbacks their staff are experiencing. And the grief of change will be exacerbated or alleviated depending upon whether the change is voluntarily or internally motivated (e.g., changing a job or life situation) versus imposed (e.g., caused by a management action). The COVID-19 pandemic is a tragic example of stresses on individuals and stresses on health care systems and practices that can cause grief responses in people.

PREPARING FOR CHANGE

At this point, you may be realizing that change management, together with decision-making and team building, share many attributes. They require planning, analytics, building of alliances, learning, input, and follow-up. Such planning is not amenable to a "trust me, I'm a doctor, I know what to do" approach. Not to say that emotional thoughts, gut reactions, and confidence are not part of change management, but these need to be tempered by scrutiny and challenging why you feel a particular way. You need to understand what unintended consequences there may be and how to respond to both those and to the expected disruptions the change will bring.

There is another cliché: "I couldn't lose control because I never had it." Being a cliché, though, doesn't mean it can't contain at least some truth. Along with understanding expected and unintended consequences, we should be prepared for losing, and then regaining, control of the situation. I like to say that once you create instability (through change) in an environment or situation, you no longer can assume to have control over what's going to happen next. Instituting a new compensation model for clinicians might seem like a good idea, but what if it disadvantages your most productive clinician and she decides to leave your practice? Developing a team care model can help share workloads, but what if it disrupts long-established clinician-patient relationships? These possibilities speak to planning change that preserves what is valued, while improving upon that base.

REDEFINING THE PROBLEM

To illustrate the change management process, I'll use a common complaint heard from clinicians and from health care managers: "Too often patients don't keep their appointments." The first teaching point is that very often we try to solve a problem—create a change—from our own point of view. With this example, a patient doesn't come for an appointment, disrupting the clinician's schedule. But what if we create a solution after defining the problem differently— is the patient not getting the care they need? Here goes.

In a health care encounter, we try to solve a problem by first asking the patient, "What brings you here today?" We call this the "chief complaint." In our management role, the chief complaint is that patients frequently don't come for

Very often we try to solve a problem—create a change— from our own point of view.

appointments, resulting in wasted time for the practice or health care system, which translates into lost revenue, missed care, and potentially bad health outcomes.

We'll next want to know more of the story—what are the "facts," the reasons for the problem? Depending upon the type of appointment and upon the type of practice, the "no-show" rate may equal 10–40 percent of appointments (lower end for specialty and hospital care, higher end for outpatient primary care). Clinicians often blame the patient for the problem—"they don't care, they don't respect my expertise and time." Or they blame the system—"insurance coverage makes it easy for patients to skip appointments; my office or facility doesn't do enough to remind patients."

Maybe, though, the reasons are more complex. The American health care system is usually very skilled at taking care of acute, severe illness and injury but has a tremendous deficit in both preventive care and the management of chronic diseases. When we look at the bundle of recommended preventive services, only a quarter of people are up to date. Looking at individual services, even for the most important, such as influenza vaccine, mammograms for breast cancer, and screening for colon cancer, the numbers are rarely better than 70 percent. The term we often use is actually 70 percent "compliance"—but this immediately puts the blame on the consumers/patients and assumes a certain set of solutions. What about chronic disease treatment, such as for hypertension (high blood pressure)? Fewer than half of Americans with this condition have their blood pressure adequately treated (controlled), despite our mega-cost system and there being at least sixty different drugs for the condition. Why? Either the patient has not been diagnosed (and may not know themselves that they have high blood pressure) or they are not treated to the appropriate outcome level.

Is it possible that our chief complaint is not just because of how the patient behaves but also has something to do with our entire approach to health care? Either way, from the point of view of both the "system" and the "consumer," there is a deficit, a condition that we would like to change.

Next, let's try to understand how we got to the current state of affairs. How have you been dealing with this issue until now? In the change process, this is where you may begin to encounter denial, anger, and depression. We might deny there is a problem, think that there is no solution, or that a fix is too hard, so why bother? Here are a few examples of that thinking and behavior from the clinician or system side:

- "We tried to fix this before and it was a waste of time." This presumes a few things: The solution(s) selected were appropriate, the planning and communication were good (including understanding the views and roles of all parties), and the present situation closely mirrors the past.

163

- "They (the consumers/patients) just don't care." (Have we asked them if they do, and have we included them in the change?)

- "We're different— things others do won't work here."

- "I don't have the time or energy to try to fix this."

- "I'm doing everything right." Or, "We've always done it this way." "It's not my fault, so why should I suffer."

What if we ask the patient why he/she didn't keep an appointment? Surprisingly this has rarely been done, but when it has, the answer often is not a lack of respect or caring. In the section called "Engaging the Change Process" that follows soon, you will find an important list of all the reasons I've encountered for why patients have missed appointments.

There are challenges for both the medical practice and the patients and not over-simplifying the "fault," and therefore the solutions, is key.

THE CONTEXT OF THE CHANGE PROCESS

Next let's take a look at the social context, the bigger picture, surrounding our dilemma. Is there something in the outside world or in our belief systems that is contributing to the problem? Not an insignificant portion of the time, the reasons for failure of a system, a solution, or a change process are rooted in assumptions, sometimes subconscious, about the people involved. Clinicians may not recognize the impact of the social determinants of health or the limitations of health insurance coverage, such as high out-of-pocket expenses for routine care and medications. Patients may feel their clinician does not respect cultural differences and lacks respect or understanding for their conceptions of wellness and disease. They may have had negative experiences from previous encounters with the health care system. These can include a failure to communicate in a common language, whether it be "foreign" as usually defined, or by using health care jargon that lay people do not easily understand. Some of the fear patients have may be a result of how their family or community have been treated in the past. Many times, I've been reminded that distrust by the Black community of institutional and individual health care providers goes back at least to the experimentation of the Tuskegee Study. It began in the 1930s and continued to the 1970s, denying many the known and effective treatment for syphilis.

In the traditional medical history, the patient is asked a long list of questions, called the review of systems. For the change process, let's think of the review of systems as our way of learning as much about the problem at hand, and how it affects all concerned.

This might include data that are more instructive than anecdotes might be. Since perception strongly influences our sense of reality, we will remember individual (often adverse) events and extrapolate them to a broader, and future, expectation. If individuals in some socio-economic group or type of insurance coverage (often Medicaid or the uninsured are "blamed") have not kept appointments in the past, it is easy for us to think and/or feel that that applies to entire groups of people. Data, both before and after a change, can help us know where to focus our efforts. They can also help us design population-specific solutions (e.g., for young, or working age, or lower-income parents).

It's also important not to think of the health care system and the consumer/patient population as adversaries. We can make the effort to see where interests may be aligned. The weekend hours example from the previous chapter on decision-making illustrates this. By having Saturday morning hours that can accommodate young parents and families, we also helped clinicians and staff who themselves found weekends better for their schedules. Maybe the medical practice has other barriers, intentional or not, that prevent patients from getting appointments that meet their needs. This could be clinician schedules not being available far enough in advance for routine follow-up care and/or limited phone or internet access for appointment scheduling.

I was once asked to consult for a primary care practice in an academic medical center. Patients were complaining about the difficulty in getting routine appointments. The reason: The schedules were only available one month in advance! Why? The clinicians wanted to maintain flexibility to take time off whenever they wanted and they wouldn't give the staff their vacation schedules. The "change" wasn't rocket science. Time-off requests would now be required six months in advance. The first week of every month was held unscheduled until one month before. If the time off wasn't needed by the clinician in that month, the schedule was opened for patients. If the clinician needed time off that month, patients already scheduled could be more easily shifted into the held week. In the past, if a patient appointment was canceled, there had been no open time to give them. The reason for patient complaints, for lack of access to care, and for patients needing to settle for inconvenient appointments that were often canceled was not on the patients; it was a clinician and system problem.

Another story, not specifically about the change process, shows how cultural differences can interfere with the basic access to, and use of, appointments. Early in my primary care career, I found I had a growing number of Asian Indians in my patient panel. I assumed this was because I was developing a good reputation for the care I was providing and word was spreading in the close-knit immigrant community. I asked one of my Indian patients what he thought—he told me that in India, engineers are highly respected, maybe more so than physicians. Many of the local immigrants were engineers, as was he. My biography mentioned my under-graduate degree in engineering. Hence my "instant" acceptance by the community.

I took care of the husband (this engineer) and his wife, and both sets of their parents, who were not fluent in English. I once needed to evaluate the elderly mother for pelvic and abdominal pain, but she refused an exam. My patient, the engineer, told me that for her to agree, he, her son-in-law, needed to be with her. I told him that was not going to happen. It wasn't how we did things; couldn't his wife come? No, it had to be him. Only after I agreed to their terms, was I able to go forward with the needed care. It was a vivid example of how a lack of understanding and acceptance of different cultures can lead to missed opportunities. We needed to change our ways; not they, theirs. They weren't challenging me but helping me understand the importance of respecting cultural differences.

ENGAGING THE CHANGE PROCESS

It's easy to impose your own experiences and biases (conscious or not) upon a change or decision process, and you'll want to discipline yourself from rushing to judgment and to solutions. You probably already know enough to think you know the answers. Indeed, some studies suggest that in the clinical setting, up to 90 percent of diagnoses are made just from hearing about the problem, before any physical examination or testing has even taken place. But as both clinicians and managers, we need to challenge those first impressions.

The earlier you engage with the people doing the work and the people who are impacted by the care received, the more support you are offering them in what may be a difficult change. Being able to share goals and even have staff (and sometimes consumers) contribute to defining those goals and to propose solutions, will allow them to reestablish some sense of control over their own work and lives.

A caveat, though, is that you can't allow them to control you. In a change process, there can be a fair amount of denial, anger, blaming, and self-interest. Remember that leadership is making it easier for others to be successful. It is not getting people to like you (hopefully they will, or will at least respect you and what you're trying to accomplish). Do not start a change process unless you are prepared to follow it through to fruition. You do not want to be insincere, to create angst without ultimately making progress. The end result may not look like what you had envisioned, but it should be an improvement, and maybe even a foundation for future efforts.

Go to the practice sites and see how things really work, talk to staff and customers. Maybe design and run some pilots. How about getting some data? Data can be a double-edged sword. Yes, we want to know the status of the current appointment system, studies that have been done in your organization or published in the literature, and patient/consumer surveys. The other "edge of the sword"—data are often not perfect, or perfectly relevant, for the problem being worked on. There will likely be a time in one of your change efforts when you will need to acknowledge that imperfection and move forward.

We are not looking just for answers, but for workable solutions. We may conclude that the reasons behind a problem are multi-factorial and the changes needed are many. For management challenges, those solutions probably include establishing supportive systems and helping people to be successful within those systems.

Here's what an assessment of patients not coming for appointments might look like:

- The cost of coming to an appointment is too high. The patient is embarrassed to tell the practice they can't afford the care, so they avoid the encounter.

- The patient can't get off from work, or can't afford to miss work, or can't get child care.

- The patient tried to keep the appointment but had transportation problems.

- The patient forgot the appointment.

- The patient did not follow through on the instructions from the last visit (testing, medications) and doesn't want to have that discussion with the clinician.

- The appointment was made so far in advance that the problem resolved on its own. Or the patient found someone who could see them sooner and didn't inform the practice.

- The practice staff, unintentionally or intentionally, gave an appointment that was not convenient or timely for the patient.

- The patient did not realize the importance of keeping the appointment for her/his own health care needs; the clinician had not taken the time to explain why follow-up care is needed, why it's done at certain intervals, and what will be done at the next appointment.

- The patient did not realize the impact on the practice of missing the appointment.

- Clincians and staff did not make it easy for the patient to communicate with them, so there was little way for her/him to ask questions or to cancel/reschedule. Maybe there are long waits on the phone, no phone access during lunch (when the patient is free to call from work), unhelpful phone staff, or a hard-to-use patient portal.

- The patient doesn't care what the practice feels. Maybe the patient doesn't think the practice cares about her/him.

Is this an exhausting list or what? I'm sure, though, that I've left out a number of possibilities. But there should be enough here to help us understand that the causes may not be simple or singular, and therefore, the solutions will not be either.

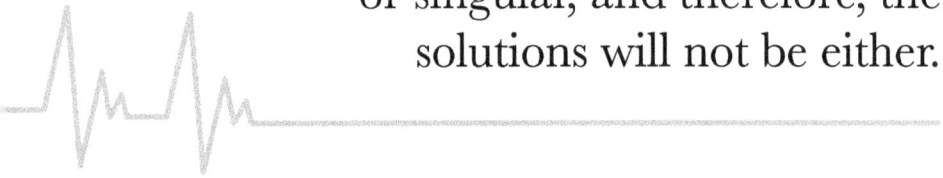

> The causes may not be simple or singular, and therefore, the solutions will not be either.

RESISTANCE TO CHANGE AND AGENTS OF CHANGE

To emphasize again, unless we look at all sides of the issue, and get multiple inputs of opinions, advice, and data, it will be difficult to change to a future state that works for all concerned. Here is a reality: Resistance to change is not futile and will quickly derail efforts to implement and manage the new state. The resistance can be active, or it can just be the elasticity that brings human beings back to the "way it always was," which generally is easier to accept and creates less tension. Just as statistics are said to regress to the mean, human behavior will regress to that of the past. Entropy, that force that follows a gradual and inexorable path to disorder, will be played out by humans as they fall back upon familiar, even if less perfect, behaviors and systems.

In our change process, we want to finalize our ideas for the future state, develop pathways and timelines to get there, build coalitions, identify change leaders. Uh, what's that last one? Aren't you as the leader/manager controlling the change? If you think so, you've missed some of the earlier points in this book. Yes, the change process may often be initiated by senior leaders, but it won't succeed unless it's owned by those who need to live with it. Even in response to an externally imposed crisis (a pandemic?), for which senior leaders will need to move quickly and rally the troops, it's better to have the change implemented by the team than imposed upon it (unless the boat is literally sinking, in which case the team should have been part of designing the abandon-ship drill). Sometimes the change will also involve things the organization's leadership needs to do differently. It can't be a situation of "everyone needs to change except me." That applies to everyone, really: A lot of people want change; few want to change themselves.

In any group facing a change, the largest number of folks start out in the "leave me alone" stage, consistent with the early stages of the grief process. As they progress through the process, they can be convinced one way or the other. But this group will largely be passive participants, at least early on. A smaller portion will be the "show me" folks. They're ready to take action but need to be convinced. They might already be in a sub-group that needs emotional support and then guidance and direction. Once activated, they can be real advocates for the change. They may be skeptics but not cynics. Another portion, also small, will be active resisters. These are the cynics or deniers: "Nothing can get better; you don't know what you're doing; it's not my fault." As the leader in the organization, you'll need to decide if these folks can change their behaviors (their personality may never change) and if what they contribute to the organization outweighs their current and future drag. They will need individual conversations and maybe graceful ways to leave the organization.

Usually, the smallest group includes the change agents on your staff and team. These are folks who thrive in chaos, who are always looking for ways to do better, and who can deal with uncertainty. They are often the informal leaders among the staff and are respected for their attention to others. They are not only open to change, they focus on results, and are effective listeners and communicators. They are the folks who the passive group, and those who can be converted, will follow. They are people who can be tapped for "bigger" things in the future. They are often humble, not looking for the spotlight nor accolades, but can recognize that the value of their contributions is bigger than themselves as individuals.

A large primary care practice I managed decided to go through a top-to-bottom redesign of how we delivered care. The people we selected to design and manage the change were those informal leaders from all levels of the practice—receptionists, medical assistants, nurses, nurse practitioners, and physicians. Their involvement gave confidence to their coworkers that the outcome would respect the needs of the staff, patients, and entire organization. Many of those informal leaders later moved successfully into formal management and leadership roles.

PLANNING CHANGE

For a change that increases the likelihood patients come for their appointments, here's a sample plan and implementation steps:

- Have a small workgroup, including frontline staff and managers, look at the data.

- Give your change team the time to work; you may need to provide other staff to off-load the regular responsibilities of the team.

- Identify a few potential interventions, which hopefully would not include "educating" or "penalizing" patients, but that instead recognizes the need for system solutions, staff training, and consumer communication.

- Test the potential interventions with a larger group of staff and possibly with a consumer focus group.

- Select the best interventions and plan an implementation, which could be phased.

- Identify metrics for the change (e.g., fewer "no-shows," fewer complaints from consumers, more job satisfaction of frontline staff, shorter appointment wait times—since there would be fewer wasted appointment slots).

- Develop a communications strategy around the change.

- Identify role models and peer and expert trainers.

- Design a training-and-change curriculum.

- Enlist the help of other work units (hopefully they were involved from the start), such as information technology, communications, and consumer services.

- Schedule the change(s) and also the check points.

- Analyze data about progress and be prepared to make adjustments along the way.

- Seek feedback.

- Provide ongoing reports.

- Stay involved for as long as needed. Culture change will make it more likely that technical and system change will work, short- and long-term, but may take many months to develop.

In my real-life example of a large primary care practice undergoing a top-to-bottom redesign, we realized that it was the frontline team who would bear the brunt of a change in how patients were scheduled. Not only were that staff part of the learning process, of designing the solution and of its implementation, they were supported by appropriate training and staffing and weren't blamed when some things didn't go as planned. We realized they were so important to the ongoing success of the work, and to the culture change, that we trained the frontline staff and the clinicians together. That in itself was an important step in changing the culture—being sure every team member knew the challenges that others faced every day.

As you can see, change is resource intensive. That's why I wholeheartedly agree with the commentators who say that the time to make changes is while things are going well in your organization. That's when you can invest in your staff and in solutions, in a thoughtful way, to make things better for the future. It's when you can make even incremental improvements that build upon something that is already good. If staff

The time to make changes is while things are going well in your organization.

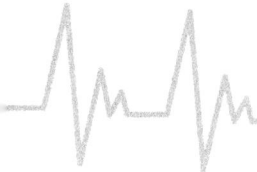

are stressed and patients are unhappy and complaining, it's hard to have the energy, time, resources, and management credibility to invest in a successful change process

From the number of words dedicated to change management, you might conclude that this is the most important part of being a leader. After all, if everything works perfectly, if there were no problems or unexpected challenges, then there would be little need for leaders and managers. "Every system is perfectly designed to get the results it gets." This quote is often attributed to Dr. Don Berwick, the founder of the Institute for Healthcare Improvement. To me, this means that to continually get better, we need to continually look at our systems, both in patient care and in how practices and health systems operate. By doing so, we will better understand that the daily work of leadership and management exists to help create an environment in which others can be successful. It achieves this goal by providing the tools that empower people to design, manage, implement, and further systematic change.

Now, I don't believe that all problems are purely system related and don't involve people themselves. At the very least, we need to be sure staff are fully able to work within a system. But there are some people who are just not good at what they do, and you'll need to decide if they can be helped. There are some people who are skilled and knowledgeable and are still not a good fit for a role or system. Can they become a better fit and are they willing to try (remember the spectrum of how people respond to change)? A central tenet of system change is to make it easier for people to do the right thing. This applies in patient care (how is it easiest for patients to make and change appointments; how is it easiest for a patient to get preventive screenings?), and it applies to management (how can we set up a scheduling system for the staff to quickly and accurately choose the right appointment for a patient?).

Change is exceptionally important. It's part of the bigger whole and cannot be separated from the other leadership and management skills. And those skills are set upon the foundation of developing and having the personal insights and attributes that allow you to be effective, efficient, and sincere when you work with others.

A central tenet of system change is to make it easier for people to do the right thing.

CHANGE MANAGEMENT TAKEAWAYS

- Change is necessary and unavoidable. People change, the outside environment changes, technologies change. Systems need to change voluntarily or need to change to adapt to new realities.

- Change is one of the biggest responsibilities and challenges of leadership and management—it is complex.

- Almost any change will be resisted by normal human beings. And resistance will often be successful.

- Be exceptionally planful when it comes to change, including the process by which it will be pursued.

- Even after initial implementation, there needs to be work to maintain, and adjust, the change.

- Coming back to the mantra attributed to President Barack Obama—"better is good"—the change you make may not be perfect, nor exactly what you want, but improvement now puts you on the path for more improvement later.

CONCLUSIONS

In my career as a practicing physician, manager, and then leader, I saw many styles and strategies of management and leadership. I saw bighearted, smart, hardworking people fail. In many cases, that failure was due to a lack of preparation or not taking the time to learn necessary skills. Sometimes their passion to do good caused conflict with someone else who was just as passionate but had different priorities or ways of getting things done. More than once, I saw someone voluntarily, or not, move on to other organizations, not always for the benefit of all concerned. By understanding how we can fail, we can better know how we can be successful.

In any leadership and management situation, there are ever so many things that can go wrong. Sometimes everything has been done just "right," but there is a bad or undesired outcome. Sometimes the outcome is great despite the underlying approach being awful. Sometimes there is more than one "right" way of doing things—there is not a "silver bullet" that fixes everything. The task I've undertaken, and the task for those who aspire to serve as leaders and managers, is to develop the personal attributes and to learn the appropriate skills, to increase the chances of success for those they care for, for those they work with, and for themselves.

I don't want to leave the impression that those trained

in and practicing health care start off with a deficit in their chances for leadership and management success. However, we need to be aware that sometimes our greatest strength will also be our greatest weakness. People who become health care clinicians are very often compassionate, passionate, thoughtful, analytic, hardworking, and perseverant. Those strengths are a boon to leadership and management. Those attributes can also make a person less tolerant of others, want to go it alone, and to lead while expecting others to simply follow. Clinicians are very often highly efficient. But that is not the same as being effective. As we've related, we can be good at getting things done, but maybe they weren't the right things to do, or maybe they turned out well despite a poorly thought-out but efficient process.

A few other examples: Both leaders and clinicians need to have the confidence that they can, and do, make the correct decisions. Otherwise, they can be paralyzed by fear of making a decision, not be able to complete a task and clear their mind for the next one, and not be able to rest calmly at night. We've all been in the presence of the highly confident person. However, when that confidence becomes hubris, when it strangles out humility and stifles the ability to learn, what has been an almost necessary strength will become a liability in the management of patients, teams, and organizations.

Similarly, an incredibly smart person for whom things come easily, may not appreciate the process and struggle that others may go through to do their jobs and to get through life. That strength can seem to others to be a lack of empathy, or even arrogance.

The highly analytic, organized person can efficiently make plans. But that strength will bring more value when empathy for the human element—understanding how those plans affect others—is taken into account and truly understood. The clinician who has been trained to be able to depersonalize in response to patient suffering can seem to remain calm and rational in tense situations. But this "cool cucumber" may seem uncaring and may be keeping too much emotion inside for the well-being of themselves and those around them.

"THE PERFECT IS THE ENEMY OF THE GOOD"

How do you interpret this saying? Some people look at it as meaning we should not settle for what is merely good but should keep pushing until we achieve perfection. To a clinician, for whom making a mistake can be tantamount to making humans suffer, it is understandable to want to get things right. But in management (and sometimes also in clinical practice) that can be dysfunctional. To me, and to many others who've written about management, this saying instead means that sometimes things aren't yet perfect, but they're worth doing nonetheless. This applies to decision-making, change management, and a host of other leadership and management challenges. Yes, don't settle for a new hire who clearly won't improve your team. But don't pass up someone because they don't fit all your criteria. Don't put aside a solution that will help many, even if there is more to be done. Future improvement is made easier by present successes.

A last story, that encapsulates the work of management: At one time I was the adult medicine chief of a multispecialty university practice. We realized that our patients were not getting their preventive health screenings at a rate close to what we all agreed was acceptable. It generally was below 50 percent on the common measures of breast, colon, and cervical cancer screening. Adult medicine included internal medicine and family medicine specialists. There was also an ob-gyn department. Some men received care from internal medicine physicians (internists), some from family medicine docs. About half of the women in the practice got their care from internal medicine and family medicine, the others from ob-gyn. What did this have to do with the poor performance on lifesaving preventive measures? Well, each specialty blamed one of the other specialties for the deficit—"of course we know how to care for ___" (fill in the blank). And the professional organizations for each specialty

Future improvement is made easier by present successes.

(the American College of Physicians, for internists; the American College of Obstetricians and Gynecologists; and the American Association of Family Practice) did not agree on the guidelines on how often many preventive measures should be performed.

Here's how we approached the issue:

- We all agreed our performance overall was a problem if viewed from the point of view of those we provided care for. No matter what guideline was used, being below 50 percent was way too low.

- We agreed to look at our screening data about our population of young women for cervical cancer, older women for breast cancer, and men and women over fifty for colon cancer. What was really going on, not who was at fault?

- We found that patients were indeed being differently treated depending upon what type of physician they were seeing. Women seeing an ob-gyn clinician were more likely to have cervical and breast screening (70% or more) than if they saw an internist or family physician (about 40%). Women seeing an ob-gyn for their regular primary care were very unlikely to have colon cancer screening (20–30%), compared to if they saw another type of primary care physician (50–60%).

- With facts in hand, we were able to make rational, pragmatic, changes. We agreed on a "least common denominator" approach. Maybe an individual clinician believed
the appropriate screening interval was one year, or maybe
two years, but we all could accept that it was no more than
two years. Doing too much preventive screening seemed
not to be our problem. So we all agreed screening could be
every one year, but needed to be at least every two years,
and designed our guidelines, patient materials and education, and outreach efforts accordingly.

- We also agreed that every specialty was responsible for the
screening of every patient it encounters. It was no longer
good enough for an ob-gyn to tell a 55-year-old woman
to make an appointment for an internist to arrange a
colonoscopy. The clinician and her staff were responsible
for being sure it was scheduled. It was no longer okay
for an internist to tell a 35-year-old woman to go to the
ob-gyn department for a pap smear (or for a 55-year-old
to schedule a mammogram and breast exam). Either the
adult medicine clinician did it herself or himself, or they
and their staff were responsible for getting it scheduled.

This was a case of good, smart people, practicing in a traditional way and doing bad things. By helping them see how
patients were being impacted, changing the system expectations and operations, and enlisting the patient population to

understand and expect certain care, we were able to move our screening rates to over 60 percent (and rising).

As a clinician who is a manager and/or a leader, or as a manager and/or leader of clinicians, take the time to understand yourself and the special personalities, knowledge, responsibilities, and experiences of health care. Look into yourself and into others to understand strengths and weaknesses. Realize that change is possible, including that of yourself and others, and takes insight, planning, and inherent qualities. It also takes the learning and relearning of management and leadership skills.

As Dr. Jerome Groopman has written, "Medicine is not an exact art. There's lots of uncertainty, always evolving information, much room for doubt. The most dangerous people are the ones who speak with total authority and no room for error."[42]

AFTERWORD

As you've come this far in reading you might be thinking, "Why, this is all common sense." And if that's the case, good for you. Then what we've discussed is a review for you and may serve to reinforce what you already know and make it fresher and more relevant to your day-to-day efforts.

But to be clear, common sense is not a value-less attribute. It is not "common," and to make "sense," it needs to be informed by character. It needs to be cultivated, shaped by experience (both good and bad), and to evolve. To the clinician, and to those who lead and manage clinicians, "common sense" needs values.

To illustrate this point, here is an example from the non-health care world:

In 2020, the United States Federal government reinstated a policy that allows hunters in Alaska to use donuts coated with bacon fat to lure bears to shoot for sport. Some might say it's common sense that this is "unfair" and "inhumane."

To the clinician, and to those who lead and manage clinicians, "common sense" needs values.

Others might question the sense of attributing rights to animals. To people this was an argument on values, of rights. To the bears, it was life and death.

"Common sense" is also informed by knowledge and understanding. That is, it is not passed to us in a final, immutable form. It evolves over time as we learn and have new experiences, until it becomes wisdom. Here is another example, contemporary to this writing, which is related to health care:

We were recently in the midst of a global COVID-19 pandemic. People were desperate to find a prevention and a cure. Some had suggested using drugs commonly used for malaria. A politician said, "What the hell do you have to lose?" He inferred that common sense would have it that it's better to do something than nothing. But learning and scientific knowledge would suggest otherwise. Treatments can have side effects that can be worse than the disease. For the patient, what they "have to lose" is delaying doing something more likely to help by using a treatment that could make them sicker.

For our society there is also a reason not to just try something. It's the opportunity cost of spending time and money on a treatment with a low probability of helping,

"Common sense" is also informed by knowledge and understanding.

while neglecting other, more likely, interventions. While our government was spending money on millions of doses of a drug (including exporting it to other countries) and taking the time of our researchers, they were delaying other investigations. And they made those drugs harder to get for those who really needed them.

So we see that both our values and our knowledge inform our "sense." Hopefully, in these pages you've gained some knowledge and understand how important your values are as an underpinning to leadership and management. How humility, listening, and being inclusive empower you.

Character is the companion of common sense; it too is molded by our experiences and learning. It is good if you come to leadership and management, and to health care, with a character that will serve you well. As with "sense," it is something that will, and should, evolve over time and can be cultivated actively (do not assume you can passively osmose yourself into success).

As I said, this afterword was written during a pandemic. At this time, many commentators referenced the novel *The Plague*, by Albert Camus. Published in 1947, it is set in the Algerian city of Oran—Algeria at that time was a French colony. (There was not actually an infectious plague in Oran at that time. It is said that Camus based his plot on past bubonic plague or cholera epidemics, or maybe even on the Nazi occupation of France.) The main protagonist of the story is a physician, Dr. Rieux. When asked how he can

Character is the companion of common sense.

persevere with so much suffering and death, and told that he is a hero, Rieux tells us: "There's no question of heroism in all this. It's a matter of common decency. That's an idea which may make some people smile, but the only means of fighting a plague is common decency."

Doesn't that sound a bit like character—humility and self-sacrifice, in the service of others?

NOTES

Chapter One: Management, Leadership, and Supervision—What's in a Name?

1. Bill Bradley, *Values of the Game* (New York: Artisan Press, 1998).

2. "Casey Stengel." https://caseystengel.org/wp-content/uploads/2010/11/stengel_brochure.pdf (accessed Sept. 11, 2023).

3. Carl Larson and Frank LaFasto, *TeamWork* (Newbury Park, California: SAGE Publications, 1989).

4. Jay Walker, "Need a Manager? I'm Not Your Guy," interview by Adam Bryant, *New York Times,* June 18, 2017.

Chapter Three: Why Physician Managers Fail

5. Bill Moyers, interview by Studs Terkel, March 2, 1993, *Voices of our Time*, Chicago Historical Society.

6. Stephen Dubner, "Why Are There So Many Bad Bosses?" March 2, 2022, in *Freakonomics Radio*, produced by Ryan Kelley, *Freakonomics* podcast, 24:50, https://freakonomics.com/?s=why%20are%20there%20so%20many%20bad%20bosses

7. Rushworth Kidder, *How Good People Make Tough Choices* (New York: Harper Perennial, rev. ed. 2009).

8. Lao Tzu, *The Tao Te Ching*, 6th Century, BCE.

9. Benedict Carey, "Be Humble, and Proudly, Psychologist Says," *New York Times*, October 21, 2019.

10. Daryl Tongeren, et al, "Humility," *Current Directions in Psychological Science* (July 2, 2019).

11. Martin M. Broadwell, "Teaching for Learning," *The Gospel Guardian* (February 20, 1969), *https://www.words-fitlyspoken.org/gospel_guardian/v20/v20n41p1-3a.html*

12. Stephen Dubner, "Hacking the World Bank (Update), Interview with Jim Yong Kim," January 12, 2019, in *Freakonomics Radio*, produced by Greg Rosalsky, *Freakonomics* podcast, 33:55, https://freakonomics.com/podcast/hacking-the-world-bank/

13. Robert Keidel, *Game Plans* (New York: Dutton Adult, 1985).

14. Richard Frankel and Terry Stein, "Getting the Most Out of the Clinical Encounter: The Four Habits," *The Journal of Medical Practice Management* vol. 16(4), (January 2001): 184–191.

15. Howard Beckman and Richard Frankel, "The Effect of Physician Behavior on the Collection of Data," *Annals of Internal Medicine* vol. 101 (November 1984): 692–696.

16. Jennifer Fong Ha, Dip Surg Anat, and Nancy Longnecker, "Doctor-Patient Communication: A Review," *The Ochsner Journal* vol. 10 (Spring, 2010): 38–43.

17. Personal communication from Kaiser Permanente.

18. Edward de Bono, *Lateral Thinking: Creativity Step by Step* (New York: HarperCollins, 2015).

19. Dara Sorkin, Israel de Alba, and Quyen Ngo-Metzger, "Racial/Ethnic Discrimination in Health Care," *Journal of General Internal Medicine* vol.25(5) (May 2010): 390–396; Sara E. Erickson, et al. "Effect of Race on Asthma Management and Outcomes," *Archives of Internal Medicine* vol. 16717 (September 2007): 1846–1852; Jessica D. Albano et al., "Cancer Mortality in the United States by Education Level and Race," *Journal of the National Cancer Institute* vol. 99(18) (September 2007): 1384–1394; Peter B. Bach et al., "Primary Care Physicians Who Treat Blacks and Whites," *New England Journal of Medicine* vol. 351(6) (August 2004): 575–584; Nancy R. Aries, "Managing Diversity: The Differing Perceptions of Managers, Line Workers, and Patients," *Health Care Management Review* vol. 29(3) (July 2004): 172–180; Robert J. Blendon et al., "Disparities in Physician Care: Experiences and Perceptions of a Multi-Ethnic America," *Health Affairs* vol. 27(2) (March–April 2008): 507–517.

20. Nick Green, "Bringing Health Food to the Masses, One Delivery at a Time," interview by David Gelles, *New York Times,* February 5, 2022.

Part II—Leadership and Management Skills

21. N. A. Stilwell et al., "Myers-Briggs Type and Medical Specialty Choice," *Teaching and Learning in Medicine* vol. 12(1) (Winter 2000): 14–20.

22. John M. Eisenberg, "Sociologic Influences on Decision-Making by Clinicians," *Annals of Internal Medicine* vol.90(6) (June, 1979): 957–964.

23. Thomas Friedman, "We Need Great Leadership Now, and Here's What it Looks Like," *New York Times*, April 21, 2020.

Chapter Four: Skill #1—Humility

24. Rob Nielsen and Jennifer A. Marrone, "Humility: Our Current Understanding of the Construct and its Role in Organizations," *International Journal of Management Reviews* vol. 20(4) (January 2018): 805–824.

25. Elizabeth J. Krumrei-Mancuso et al., "Links Between Intellectual Humility and Acquiring Knowledge," *Journal of Positive Psychology* vol. 15(2) (February 2019): 155–170.

Chapter Five: Skill #2—Building the Team

26. John Bacon, "Leadership Advice from the Coach of America's 'Worst' Hockey Team," interview by Shawna Richer, *New York Times,* January 1, 2022.

27. Tom S. Turner, *Behavioral Interviewing Guide* (Victoria, Canada: Trafford Publishing, 2004).

28. Dan Ciampa and Michael D. Watkins, *Right from the Start: Taking Charge in a New Leadership Role* (Boston: Harvard Business Review Press, 2005).

29. Marshall Goldsmith, *What Got You Here Won't Get You There* (New York: Hachette Publishing, 2007).

Chapter Seven: Skill #4—Meetings

30. Leslie A. Perlow, Constance Noonan Hadley, and Eunice Eun, "Stop the Meeting Madness," *Harvard Business Review* (July–August 2017).

31. Korn Ferry Survey, *Working or Wasting Time?,* 2019, https://www.kornferry.com/about-us/press/working-or-wasting-time.

32. George C. Herring, *America's Longest War: The United States and Vietnam 1950–1975* (New York: McGraw-Hill Publishing, 2001).

Chapter Eight: Skill #5—Critical Conversations

33. Naresh Khatri, Gordon D. Brown, and Lanis L Hicks, "From a Blame Culture to a Just Culture in Health Care," *Health Care Management Review* vol. 34(4) (October–December 2009): 312–322.

Chapter Nine: Skill #6—Negotiation

34. Gerald J. Nierenberg, *The Art of Negotiating* (New York: Cornerstone Library, 1971).

35. Roger Fisher, William L. Ury, and Bruce Patton, *Getting to Yes* (New York: Penguin Books, 2011).

36. Adam Grant, "In Negotiations, Givers are Smarter than Takers," *New York Times*, March 27, 2020. Adam Grant, *WorkLife* with Adam Grant, A TED Original Podcast, *The Science of the Deal*. March 23, 2020. Grace Rubenstein, Story Editor.

37. Stacey Sheridan, Russell Harris, and Steven Woolf, "Shared Decision Making About Screening and Chemoprevention: A Suggested Approach from the U.S. Preventive Services Task Force," *American Journal of Preventive Medicine* vol. 26(1) (January 2004): 58–66.

38. Amy Irwin et al., "Flexible Intervention to Decrease Antibiotic Overuse in Primary Care Practice," *Agency for Health Quality Research* (June 2014): 82–89, https://www.ahrq.gov/hai/patient-safety-resources/advances-in-hai/hai-article6.html

39. Mariam de la Poza Abad et al., "Prescription Strategies in Acute Uncomplicated Respiratory Infections," *JAMA Internal Medicine* vol. 176(1) (January 2016): 21–29.

Chapter Ten: Skill #7—Decision-Making

40. Shai Danzinger, Jonathan Levay, and Liora Avnaim-Pesso, "Extraneous Factors in Judicial Decisions," *Proceedings of the National Academy of Science* vol. 108 (April 26, 2011): 6889–6892.

Chapter Eleven: Skill #8—Creating the Culture

41. Marc Bard, MD, Personal communication.

Conclusions

42. Jerome Groopman, *How Doctors Think* (New York: Houghton Mifflin Company, 2007).

www.ingramcontent.com/pod-product-compliance
Lightning Source LLC
Chambersburg PA
CBHW062130020426

42335CB00013B/1168